DASH DIET COOKBOOK FOR BEGINNERS

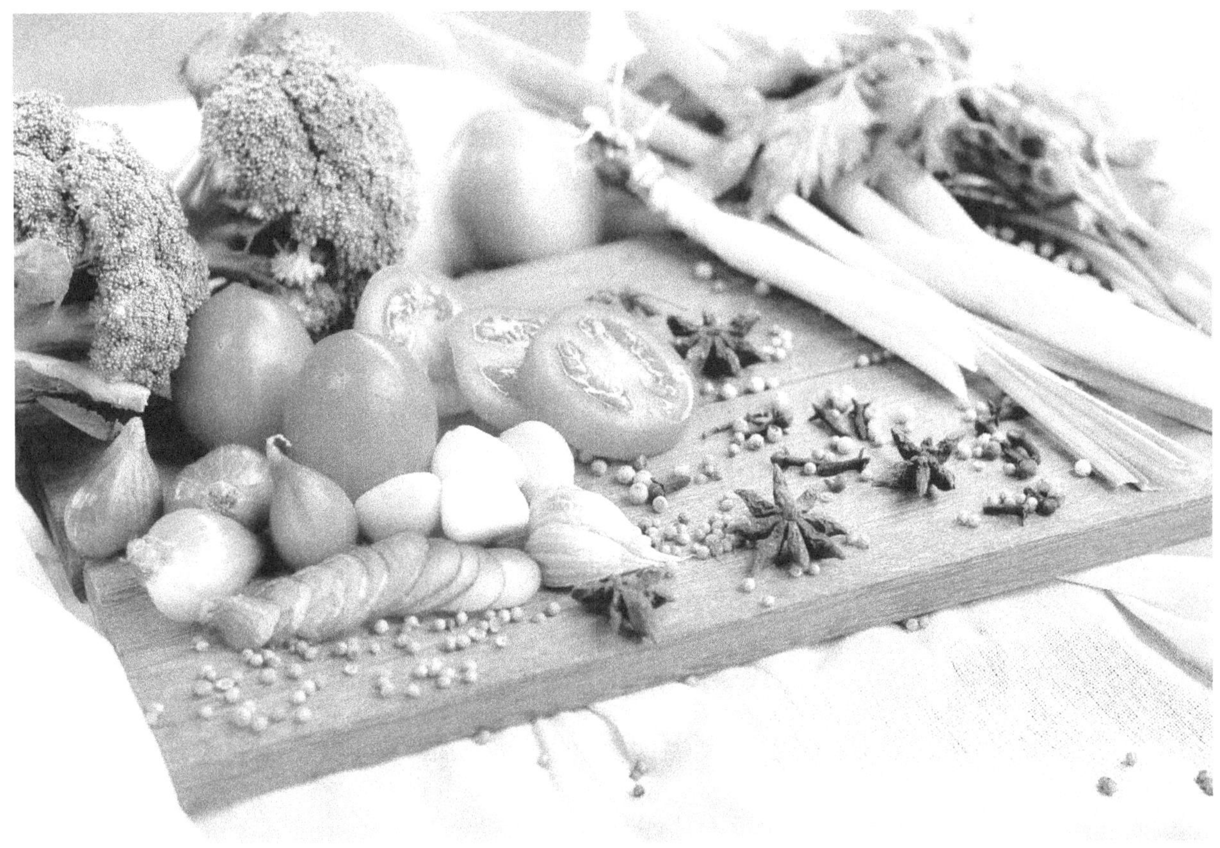

1500 Days Quick and Easy Recipes to Lower your Blood Pressure and Promote Overall Heart Health with 30 Days Meal Plan

Catherine Ellis

Copyright © 2024 by [Catherine Ellis]

SEE MORE OF MY BOOK

TYPE 2 DIABETES COOKBOOK FOR BEGINNERS

Quick, Easy, Delicious, Tasty and Nutritious Low Sugar and Low Carb Recipes with a 30 Days Meal Plan for Type 2 Diabetes

HEART HEALTHY COOKBOOK FOR BEGINNERS

Quick, Easy and Tasty Low Sodium and Low- Fat Recipes with a 30 Days Meal Plan to Manage Your Body Weight, Blood Pressure and Cholesterol Level

ANTI – INFLAMMATORY DIET COOKBOOK FOR BEGINNERS

Quick and Easy Recipes to reduce Inflammation, Healing and Boosting Immune System, improve your Health and Detoxifying your body

JUICING FOR BEGINNERS

TABLE OF CONTENT

2. Lentil Vegetable Soup

3. Brown Rice and Vegetable Stir-Fry

4. Chickpea and Spinach Curry

5. Whole Wheat Pasta Primavera

6. Black Bean and Sweet Potato Tacos

7. Quinoa Stuffed Bell Peppers

8. Barley and Vegetable Soup

9. Chickpea and Quinoa Salad

10. Brown Rice and Black Bean Burrito Bowl

CHAPTER 5

Vegetarian Recipes

Quinoa-Stuffed Bell Peppers:

Vegetable Stir-Fry with Tofu:

Mediterranean Chickpea Salad:

Spinach and Feta Stuffed Portobello Mushrooms:

Lentil and Vegetable Soup:

Vegetable and Bean Chili:

Greek Yogurt and Berry Parfait:

Whole Wheat Veggie Pizza:

Tofu and Vegetable Kabobs:

Oatmeal with Mixed Berries and Almonds:

CHAPTER 6

Vegan Recipes

1. Quinoa Vegetable Stir-Fry

2. Lentil and Vegetable Soup

3. Chickpea and Vegetable Curry

4. Spinach and Mushroom Stuffed Bell Peppers

5. Black Bean and Corn Salad

6. Mediterranean Quinoa Salad

7. Tofu and Vegetable Stir-Fry

8. Vegan Chili

9. Vegan Buddha Bowl

10. Vegan Lentil Sloppy Joes

CHAPTER 7

Poultry, Meat and Lamb Recipes

1. Grilled Lemon Herb Chicken:

2. Turkey and Quinoa Stuffed Bell Peppers:

3. Herb-Crusted Baked Salmon:

4. Mediterranean Lamb Skewers:

5. Lean Beef Stir-Fry:

INTRODUCTION

What is Dash Diet

The DASH (Dietary Approaches to Stop Hypertension) diet is a dietary approach specifically designed to help lower blood pressure. It emphasizes eating foods that are rich in nutrients such as potassium, calcium, and magnesium, which are known to help regulate blood pressure. The DASH diet also encourages reducing sodium intake, as high sodium consumption is linked to hypertension.

Key Components of Dash Diet

Emphasis on Fruits and Vegetables:

Fruits and vegetables are a great source of dietary fiber, antioxidants, and important vitamins and minerals

They are low in calories and high in nutrients, making them ideal choices for a healthy diet.

Consuming a variety of colorful fruits and vegetables provides a wide range of nutrients that support overall health and help lower blood pressure.

Inclusion of Whole Grains:

Whole grains such as brown rice, whole wheat bread, oats, barley, and quinoa are rich in fiber, vitamins, and minerals.

In addition to supporting digestive health and promoting satiety, fiber also helps control blood sugar levels

Whole grains provide sustained energy and contribute to overall heart health, making them a staple in the DASH diet.

Lean Protein Sources:

Lean protein sources include poultry (such as chicken and turkey), fish, beans, lentils, nuts, and seeds.

These protein sources are lower in saturated fat compared to red meat and processed meats, which can contribute to heart disease and high blood pressure.

Consuming lean protein supports muscle health, provides essential amino acids, and helps maintain a healthy weight.

Low-Fat Dairy Products:

Low-fat or fat-free dairy products such as milk, yogurt, and cheese are included in the DASH diet to provide calcium, potassium, and vitamin D.

Calcium and potassium play important roles in regulating blood pressure and supporting bone health.

Choosing low-fat dairy options helps reduce saturated fat intake while still obtaining essential nutrients.

Limited Sodium Intake:

The DASH diet emphasizes reducing sodium intake to help lower blood pressure and reduce the risk of heart disease.

High sodium intake is associated with hypertension, fluid retention, and increased risk of stroke.

To limit sodium intake, it's recommended to avoid processed and packaged foods high in sodium, use herbs and spices for flavoring instead of salt, and choose fresh or minimally processed ingredients.

Benefits of the Dash Diet

Lower Blood Pressure: The DASH diet is specifically designed to reduce blood pressure, making it an effective dietary approach for individuals with hypertension.

Heart Health: By emphasizing nutrient-rich foods and reducing sodium intake, the DASH diet supports heart health and reduces the risk of cardiovascular diseases such as heart attack and stroke.

Improved Cholesterol Levels: The DASH diet can help lower LDL (bad) cholesterol levels and raise HDL (good) cholesterol levels, contributing to better overall cholesterol profiles.

Weight Management: With its focus on whole foods, lean proteins, and limited processed foods, the DASH diet can aid in weight management and promote healthy weight loss.

Nutrient-Rich Diet: The DASH diet encourages the consumption of fruits, vegetables, whole grains, lean proteins, and low-fat dairy products, providing essential nutrients such as vitamins, minerals, and antioxidants.

Better Blood Sugar Control: By emphasizing whole grains, fruits, and vegetables, the DASH diet can help stabilize blood sugar levels, making it beneficial for individuals with diabetes or those at risk of developing diabetes.

Reduced Risk of Chronic Diseases: Following the DASH diet has been associated with a lower risk of chronic diseases such as type 2 diabetes, certain cancers, and kidney disease, due to its emphasis on a balanced and nutritious eating pattern.

In summary, the DASH diet offers a range of health benefits, including lower blood pressure, improved heart health, weight management support, better blood sugar control, and reduced risk of chronic diseases, making it a valuable dietary approach for overall health and well-being.

Food to Eat and Avoid in Dash Diet

Foods to Eat:

Fruits and vegetables: Packed with fiber, vitamins, and minerals

Whole grains: Brown rice, whole wheat bread, oats, quinoa.

Lean proteins: Chicken, turkey, fish, beans, lentils, nuts, seeds.

Low-fat dairy: Milk, yogurt, cheese (low-fat or fat-free).

Nuts, seeds, and legumes: Almonds, peanuts, sunflower seeds, beans, lentils.

Healthy fats: Olive oil, avocado, nuts, seeds.

Foods to Avoid or Limit:

Processed foods: Rich in harmful fats and sodium.

Red meat: Limit consumption due to its saturated fat content.

Sugary beverages: Soda, fruit juices with added sugars.

High-sodium foods: Processed meats, canned soups, salty snacks.

Sweets and desserts: Cakes, cookies, candies, pastries.

Full-fat dairy: High in saturated fats, choose low-fat or fat-free options.

By emphasizing whole, nutrient-rich foods and limiting processed and high-sodium options, the DASH diet aims to promote heart health, lower blood pressure, and support overall well-bcing.

Shopping List

Produce:

Spinach

Kale

Broccoli

Carrots

Bell peppers (variety of colors)

Tomatoes

Cucumbers

Apples

Bananas

Berries (strawberries, blueberries, raspberries)

Oranges

Lemons

Avocados

Garlic

Onions

Grains:

Whole wheat bread

Brown rice

Quinoa

Oats

Whole grain pasta

Proteins:

Chicken breasts

Turkey breast

Salmon

Tuna

Eggs

Black beans

Chickpeas

Lentils

Tofu

Dairy:

Low-fat or fat-free milk

Low-fat or fat-free yogurt

Low-fat or fat-free cheese

Cottage cheese

Nuts, Seeds, and Legumes:

Almonds

Walnuts

Peanuts

Sunflower seeds

Chia seeds

Flaxseeds

Black beans

Lentils

Healthy Fats:

Olive oil

Avocado oil

Avocados

Olives

Other:

Herbs and spices (oregano, basil, thyme, rosemary, cinnamon, cumin, paprika, etc.)

Vinegar (balsamic, apple cider, red wine)

Low-sodium soy sauce

Dijon mustard

Plain popcorn

Dark chocolate (at least 70% cocoa)

Herbal teas

Remember to prioritize fresh, whole foods and choose low-sodium options whenever possible.

It's also essential to read labels and opt for items with minimal added sugars and unhealthy fats.

This shopping list provides a good foundation for following the DASH diet and promoting heart health and overall well-being.

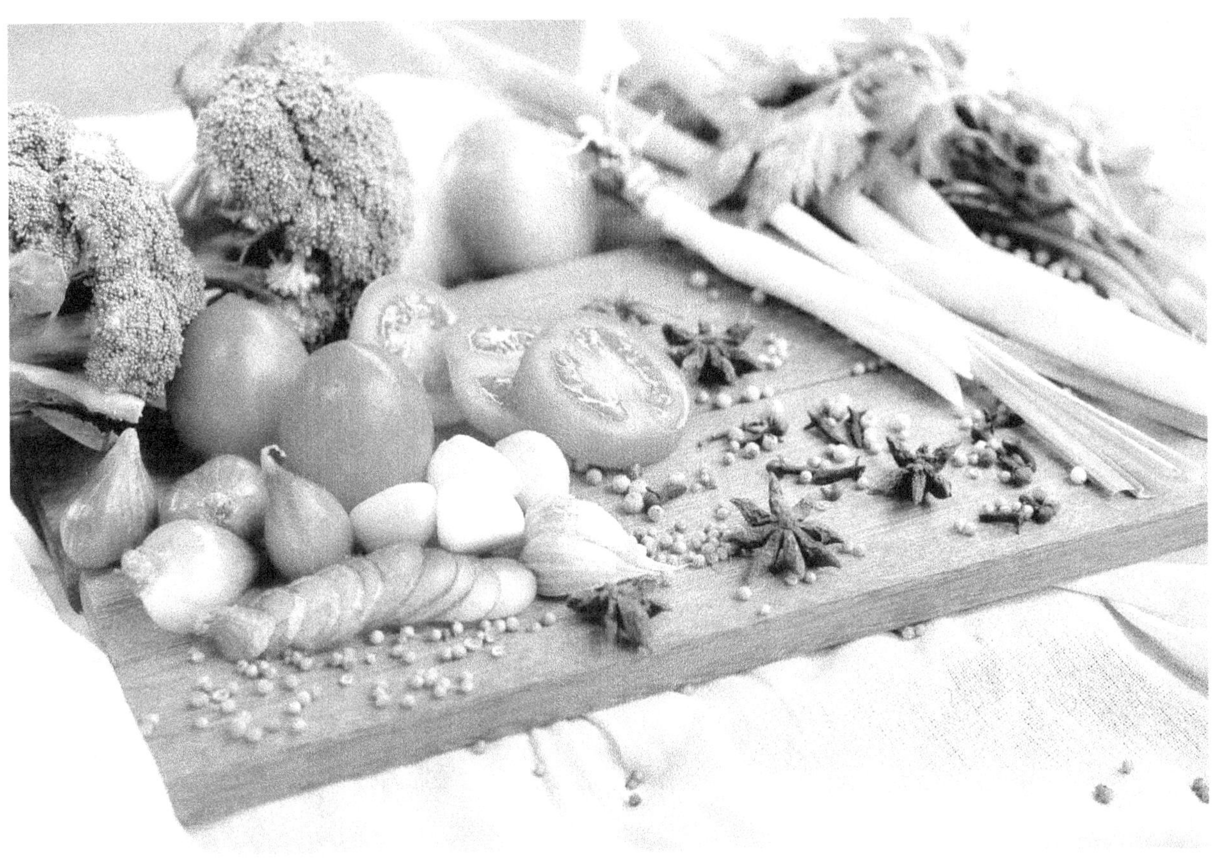

CHAPTER 1

Breakfast Recipes

Introduction:

These breakfast recipes are packed with nutrient-rich ingredients that align with the DASH diet principles. They offer a delicious and satisfying way to start your day while supporting lower blood pressure and overall heart health.

1. Avocado Toast with Poached Egg:

Ingredients:

Whole grain bread

Ripe avocado

Eggs

Lemon juice

Salt and pepper

Optional toppings: cherry tomatoes, microgreens

Instructions:

Toast the whole grain bread until golden brown.

Add the lemon juice, salt, and pepper and mash the ripe avocado. Spread it over the toasted bread.

Poach or fry an egg to your desired doneness and place it on top of the avocado spread.

Garnish with sliced cherry tomatoes and microgreens if desired.

Nutrients:

Provides fiber from whole grain bread and avocado.

Rich in healthy fats from avocado.

High in protein from eggs.

Prep Time: 10 minutes

2. Greek Yogurt Parfait:

Ingredients:

Greek yogurt (low-fat or fat-free)

Fresh berries (strawberries, blueberries, raspberries)

Granola (low-sugar)

Honey or maple syrup (optional)

Instructions:

In a glass or bowl, layer Greek yogurt, fresh berries, and granola.

Repeat layers until the glass is filled.

If desired, drizzle with maple syrup or honey.

Nutrients:

High in protein and calcium from Greek yogurt.

Rich in antioxidants and fiber from berries.

Provides whole grains and fiber from granola.

Prep Time: 5 minutes

3. Spinach and Mushroom Omelette:

Ingredients:

Eggs

Fresh spinach leaves

Mushrooms, sliced

Onion, diced

Olive oil

Salt and pepper

Optional: feta cheese

Instructions:

In a nonstick skillet, warm the olive oil over medium heat.

Sauté diced onion and sliced mushrooms until softened.

Cook the fresh spinach leaves until they wilt.

In a separate bowl, beat eggs with salt and pepper.

Pour the egg mixture into the skillet over the vegetables.

Cook until the omelette is set and the bottom has a light brown color

Fold the omelette in half and continue cooking until cooked through.

Optional: Sprinkle with crumbled feta cheese before serving.

Nutrients:

High in protein from eggs.

Provides vitamins and minerals from spinach and mushrooms.

Rich in healthy fats from olive oil.

Prep Time: 15 minutes

4. Banana Walnut Overnight Oats:

Ingredients:

Rolled oats

Unsweetened almond milk

Ripe bananas, mashed

Chopped walnuts

Cinnamon

Honey or maple syrup (optional)

Instructions:

In a jar or bowl, combine rolled oats, almond milk, mashed bananas, chopped walnuts, and a dash of cinnamon.

Stir well to combine.

Cover and refrigerate overnight.

In the morning, stir the oats mixture and add honey or maple syrup if desired.

Nutrients:

High in fiber from oats and bananas.

Provides omega-3 fatty acids from walnuts.

Rich in potassium and magnesium from bananas.

Prep Time: 5 minutes

5. Whole Grain Pancakes with Berries:

Ingredients:

Whole wheat flour

Baking powder

Salt

Eggs

Milk (low-fat or plant-based)

Vanilla extract

Fresh berries (strawberries, blueberries, raspberries)

Maple syrup or honey

Instructions:

In a mixing bowl, whisk together whole wheat flour, baking powder, and salt.

In a separate bowl, beat eggs and then stir in milk and vanilla extract.

Stirring until just blended, gradually add the wet components to the dry ingredients.

Grease or cook spray a nonstick skillet and heat it over medium heat

Pour batter onto the skillet to form pancakes.

Cook until surface bubbles appear, then turn and continue cooking until golden brown

Serve pancakes topped with fresh berries and a drizzle of maple syrup or honey.

Nutrients:

Provides whole grains and fiber from whole wheat flour.

High in protein from eggs and milk.

Rich in antioxidants and vitamins from fresh berries.

Prep Time: 20 minutes

6. Veggie Breakfast Burrito:

Ingredients:

Whole grain tortillas

Eggs

Bell peppers, diced

Onion, diced

Spinach leaves

Black beans (canned, drained and rinsed)

Avocado, sliced

Salsa or hot sauce (optional)

Instructions:

In a skillet, sauté diced onion and bell peppers until softened.

Add spinach leaves and cook until wilted.

In a separate bowl, scramble eggs and cook until set.

Warm the whole grain tortillas in the microwave or on a skillet.

Fill each tortilla with scrambled eggs, sautéed vegetables, black beans, and sliced avocado.

Roll up the tortillas to form burritos.

If desired, top with hot sauce or salsa and serve.

Nutrients:

High in protein from eggs and black beans.

Provides vitamins and minerals from vegetables.

Rich in healthy fats from avocado.

Prep Time: 15 minutes

7. Berry Spinach Smoothie:

Ingredients:

Fresh spinach leaves

Mixed berries (strawberries, blueberries, raspberries)

Banana

Greek yogurt (low-fat or fat-free)

Unsweetened almond milk

Chia seeds (optional)

Instructions:

Place spinach leaves, mixed berries, banana, Greek yogurt, and almond milk in a blender.

Blend until smooth and creamy.

If desired, add chia seeds for an extra nutritional boost and blend again briefly.

After transferring the smoothie into glasses, serve it right away.

Nutrients:

High in fiber from spinach, berries, and banana.

Provides protein and probiotics from Greek yogurt.

Rich in antioxidants and vitamins from berries.

Prep Time: 5 minutes

8. Apple Cinnamon Oatmeal:

Ingredients:

Rolled oats

Water or milk (low-fat or plant-based)

Apple, diced

Cinnamon

Honey or maple syrup (optional)

Chopped nuts (walnuts, almonds) (optional)

Instructions:

Heat up some milk or water in a pot.

Stir in rolled oats, diced apple, and a dash of cinnamon.

Reduce heat and simmer, stirring occasionally, until oats are cooked and apples are tender.

If desired, sweeten with honey or maple syrup.

Serve oatmeal hot, topped with chopped nuts if desired.

Nutrients:

High in fiber from oats and apple.

Provides vitamins and minerals from apple and cinnamon.

Optional nuts add healthy fats and protein.

Prep Time: 10 minutes

9. Smoked Salmon and Avocado Toast:

Ingredients:

Whole grain bread

Ripe avocado

Smoked salmon

Lemon juice

Salt and pepper

Optional: capers, red onion slices, dill

Instructions:

Toast the whole grain bread until golden brown.

Add the lemon juice, salt, and pepper and mash the ripe avocado

Spread it over the toasted bread.

Layer smoked salmon on top of the avocado spread.

Optional: Garnish with capers, thinly sliced red onion, and fresh dill.

Nutrients:

Provides omega-3 fatty acids from smoked salmon.

Rich in healthy fats from avocado.

High in protein and low in saturated fat from whole grain bread.

Prep Time: 10 minutes

10. Veggie Egg Muffins:

Ingredients:

Eggs

Bell peppers, diced

Spinach, chopped

Cherry tomatoes, halved

Onion, diced

Salt and pepper

Optional: shredded cheese

Instructions:

Set a muffin tin to 350°F (175°C) and preheat the oven.

In a bowl, whisk together eggs, diced bell peppers, chopped spinach, halved cherry tomatoes, diced onion, salt, and pepper.

Using a uniform pouring motion, fill each muffin cup to about 3/4 of the way to the top

Optional: Sprinkle shredded cheese on top of each muffin.

Bake the egg muffins for 20 to 25 minutes, or until they are firm and have a hint of color

Before removing from the muffin tray, let cool somewhat. Serve warm.

Nutrients:

High in protein from eggs.

Provides vitamins and minerals from vegetables.

Low in carbohydrates and suitable for a DASH diet.

Prep Time: 15 minutes

Lunch Recipes

Dietary Approaches to Stop Hypertension, or DASH, is well known for its capacity to reduce blood pressure and strengthen the heart. Here are five nutritious lunch recipes designed to support these goals, featuring wholesome ingredients and simple preparations.

1. Quinoa Salad with Chickpeas and Veggies

Ingredients:

1 cup cooked quinoa

1 can chickpeas, drained and rinsed

1 cup diced cucumbers

1 cup cherry tomatoes, halved

1/4 cup chopped parsley

2 tablespoons lemon juice

1 tablespoon olive oil

Salt and pepper to taste

Instructions:

In a large bowl, combine quinoa, chickpeas, cucumbers, tomatoes, and parsley.

In a small bowl, whisk together lemon juice, olive oil, salt, and pepper.

Drizzle the salad with the dressing, tossing to coat thoroughly

Serve chilled or at room temperature.

Nutrients: Rich in fiber, protein, vitamins, and minerals.

Prep Time: 15 minutes.

2. Grilled Salmon with Asparagus

Ingredients:

2 salmon fillets

1 bunch asparagus, trimmed

2 tablespoons olive oil

1 tablespoon lemon juice

2 cloves garlic, minced

Salt and pepper to taste

Instructions:

Preheat grill to medium-high heat.

In a small bowl, mix olive oil, lemon juice, garlic, salt, and pepper.

Brush salmon fillets and asparagus with the mixture.

Cook the salmon on the grill for 4–5 minutes on each side, or until it's done

Grill asparagus for 3-4 minutes, turning occasionally.

Serve hot.

Nutrients: High in omega-3 fatty acids, protein, and vitamins.

Prep Time: 20 minutes.

3. Turkey and Avocado Wrap

Ingredients:

4 whole-grain tortillas

8 slices turkey breast

1 avocado, sliced

1 cup baby spinach leaves

1/4 cup hummus

Instructions:

Lay tortillas flat and spread hummus evenly over each.

Layer turkey slices, avocado slices, and spinach leaves on each tortilla.

Roll tightly and cut in half.

Serve immediately or wrap tightly in foil for later.

Nutrients: Packed with lean protein, healthy fats, fiber, and vitamins.

Prep Time: 10 minutes.

4. Lentil Soup

Ingredients:

1 cup dried lentils, rinsed

1 onion, diced

2 carrots, diced

2 celery stalks, diced

4 cups low-sodium vegetable broth

2 cloves garlic, minced

1 teaspoon cumin

Salt and pepper to taste

Instructions:

In a large pot, sauté onion, carrots, and celery until softened.

Add garlic and cumin, and cook for another minute.

Stir in lentils and vegetable broth.

Bring to a boil, then reduce heat and simmer for 20-25 minutes, or until lentils are tender.

Season with salt and pepper to taste.

Serve hot.

Nutrients: High in fiber, protein, and various vitamins and minerals. **Prep Time:** 30 minutes.

5. Greek Salad with Grilled Chicken

Ingredients:

2 boneless, skinless chicken breasts

4 cups mixed salad greens

1 cucumber, sliced

1 cup cherry tomatoes, halved

1/4 cup sliced red onion

1/4 cup crumbled feta cheese

2 tablespoons olive oil

1 tablespoon red wine vinegar

1 teaspoon dried oregano

Salt and pepper to taste

Instructions:

Preheat grill to medium-high heat.

Add dried oregano, salt, and pepper to chicken breasts for seasoning.

Cook the chicken for 6–7 minutes on each side, or until it's thoroughly cooked

In a large bowl, toss salad greens, cucumber, tomatoes, red onion, and feta cheese.

In a small bowl, whisk together olive oil and red wine vinegar.

Dress salad by pouring over it and tossing to coat evenly.

Slice grilled chicken and serve over the salad.

Nutrients: Abundant in lean protein, fiber, vitamins, and minerals.

Prep Time: 25 minutes.

Dinner Recipes

Introduction:

Dinner is an essential part of the day to enjoy a nutritious meal that supports heart health and helps in lowering blood pressure. Here are five delicious DASH diet dinner recipes featuring wholesome ingredients and simple preparations to keep you on track with your health goals.

1. Baked Lemon Herb Salmon

Ingredients:

4 salmon fillets

2 tablespoons lemon juice

2 cloves garlic, minced

1 tablespoon chopped fresh dill

1 tablespoon chopped fresh parsley

Salt and pepper to taste

Instructions:

Preheat oven to 400°F (200°C).

In a small bowl, mix lemon juice, garlic, dill, parsley, salt, and pepper.

Arrange the salmon fillets on a parchment paper-lined baking pan.

Brush salmon with the lemon herb mixture.

Bake the salmon for 12 to 15 minutes, or until it is thoroughly done

Serve hot.

Nutrients: Packed with protein, important vitamins, and omega-3 fatty acids.

Prep Time: 10 minutes.

2. Quinoa Stuffed Bell Peppers

Ingredients:

Four big bell peppers, seeded and halved

1 cup cooked quinoa

1 can black beans, drained and rinsed

1 cup diced tomatoes

1/2 cup corn kernels

1/4 cup chopped cilantro

1 teaspoon cumin

Salt and pepper to taste

Instructions:

Preheat oven to 375°F (190°C).

In a large bowl, mix cooked quinoa, black beans, tomatoes, corn, cilantro, cumin, salt, and pepper.

Stuff the quinoa mixture into each side of a bell pepper.

Place stuffed peppers in a baking dish and cover with foil.

Bake peppers for 25 to 30 minutes, or until soft.

Serve warm.

Nutrients: High in fiber, protein, antioxidants, and vitamins.

Prep Time: 20 minutes.

3. Vegetable Stir-Fry with Tofu

Ingredients:

1 block tofu, cubed

2 tablespoons low-sodium soy sauce

1 tablespoon sesame oil

2 cloves garlic, minced

1 tablespoon grated ginger

Two cups of mixed veggies, including carrots, broccoli, and bell peppers

Cooked brown rice for serving

Instructions:

In a bowl, marinate tofu in soy sauce, sesame oil, garlic, and ginger for 15 minutes.

A big wok or skillet should be heated to medium heat.

Add marinated tofu and cook until golden brown, about 5 minutes.

Add mixed vegetables to the skillet and stir-fry for another 5-7 minutes, or until vegetables are tender-crisp.

Serve over cooked brown rice.

Nutrients: Packed with protein, fiber, vitamins, and minerals.

Prep Time: 20 minutes.

4. Mediterranean Chickpea Salad

Ingredients:

2 cans chickpeas, drained and rinsed

1 cucumber, diced

1 cup cherry tomatoes, halved

1/4 cup sliced red onion

1/4 cup chopped parsley

1/4 cup crumbled feta cheese

2 tablespoons olive oil

2 tablespoons lemon juice

1 teaspoon dried oregano

Salt and pepper to taste

Instructions:

Chickpeas, cucumber, tomatoes, red onion, parsley, and feta cheese should all be combined in a big bowl

In a small bowl, whisk together olive oil, lemon juice, oregano, salt, and pepper.

Drizzle the salad with the dressing, tossing to coat thoroughly

Serve chilled or at room temperature.

Nutrients: Rich in fiber, protein, healthy fats, and antioxidants.

Prep Time: 15 minutes.

5. Turkey and Vegetable Skewers

Ingredients:

2 turkey breasts, cut into cubes

2 bell peppers, cut into chunks

1 zucchini, sliced

1 red onion, cut into chunks

2 tablespoons olive oil

1 tablespoon balsamic vinegar

1 teaspoon dried thyme

Salt and pepper to taste

Instructions:

Set the grill pan or grill to medium-high heat.

Thread turkey cubes, bell pepper chunks, zucchini slices, and red onion chunks onto skewers.

In a small bowl, mix olive oil, balsamic vinegar, dried thyme, salt, and pepper.

Brush skewers with the olive oil mixture.

Grill skewers for 10-12 minutes, turning occasionally, until turkey is cooked through and vegetables are tender.

Serve hot.

Nutrients: High in lean protein, fiber, vitamins, and minerals.

Prep Time: 20 minutes.

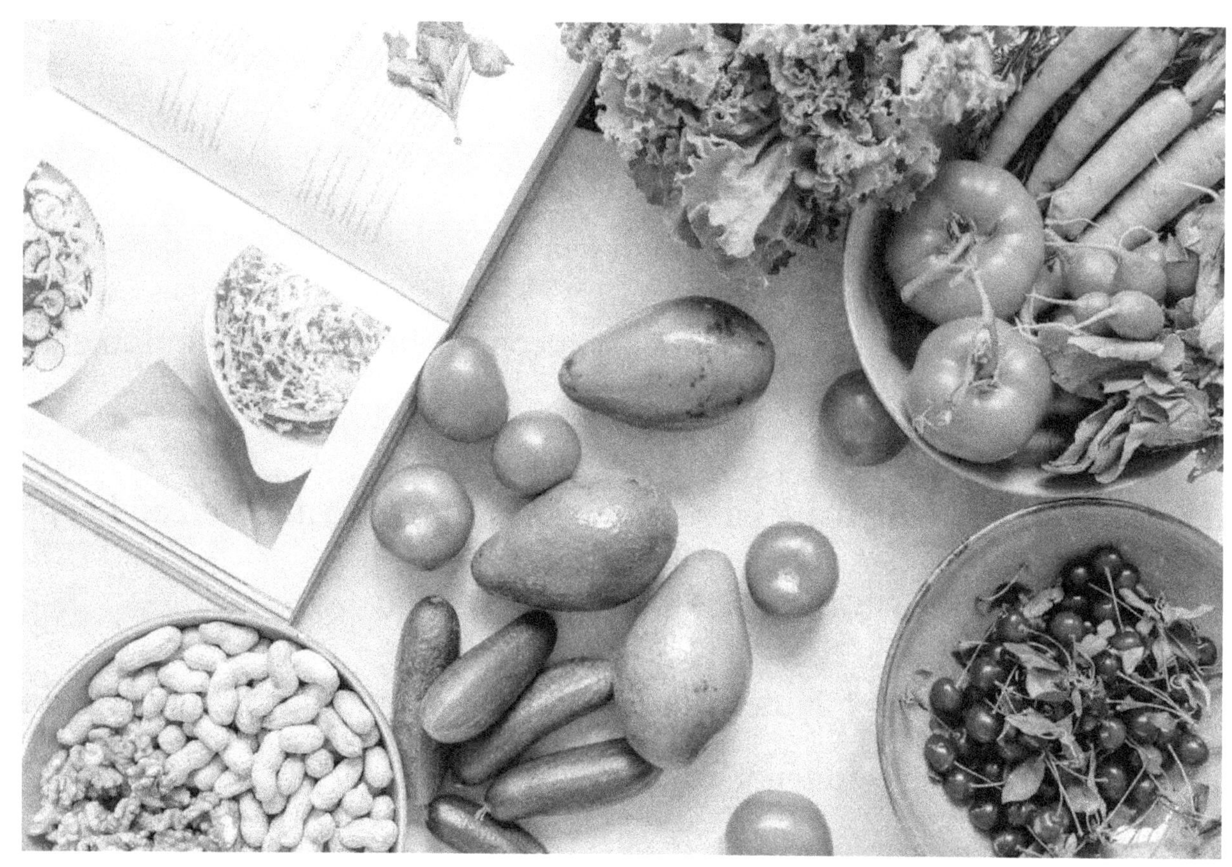

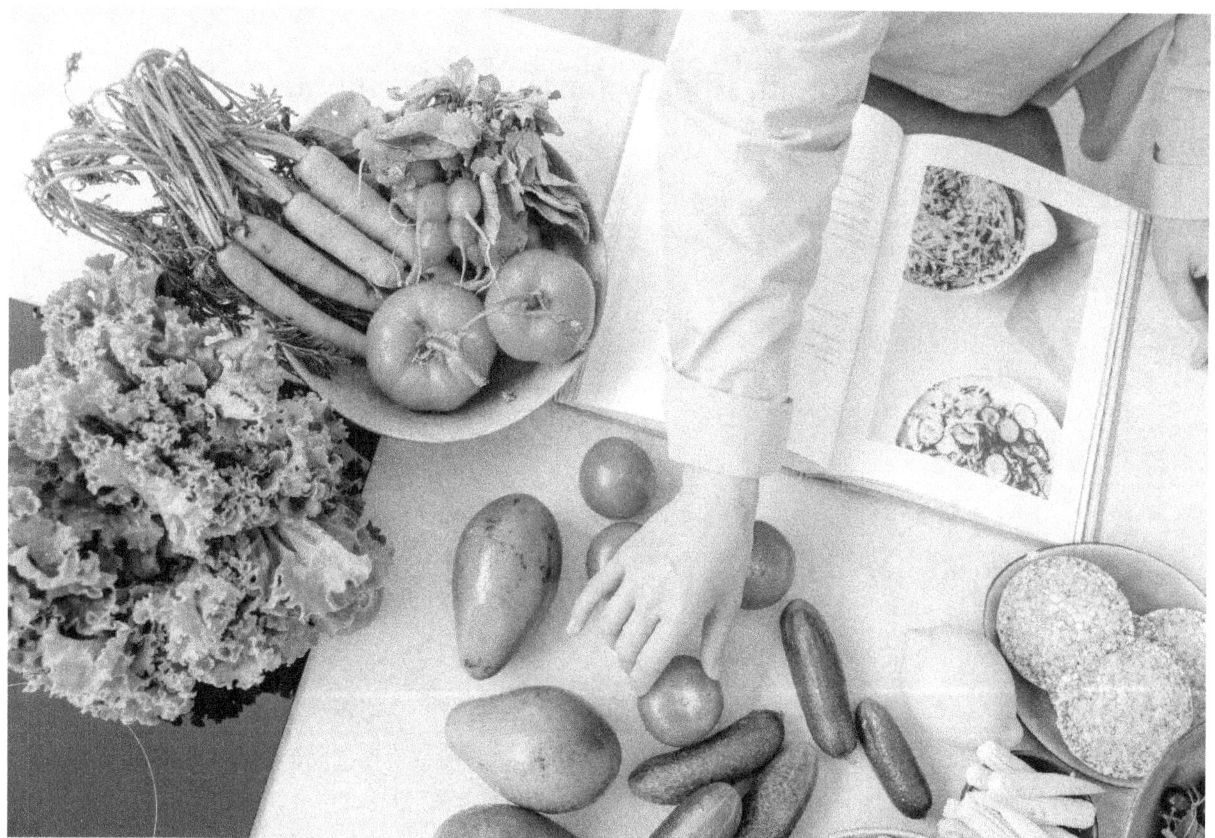

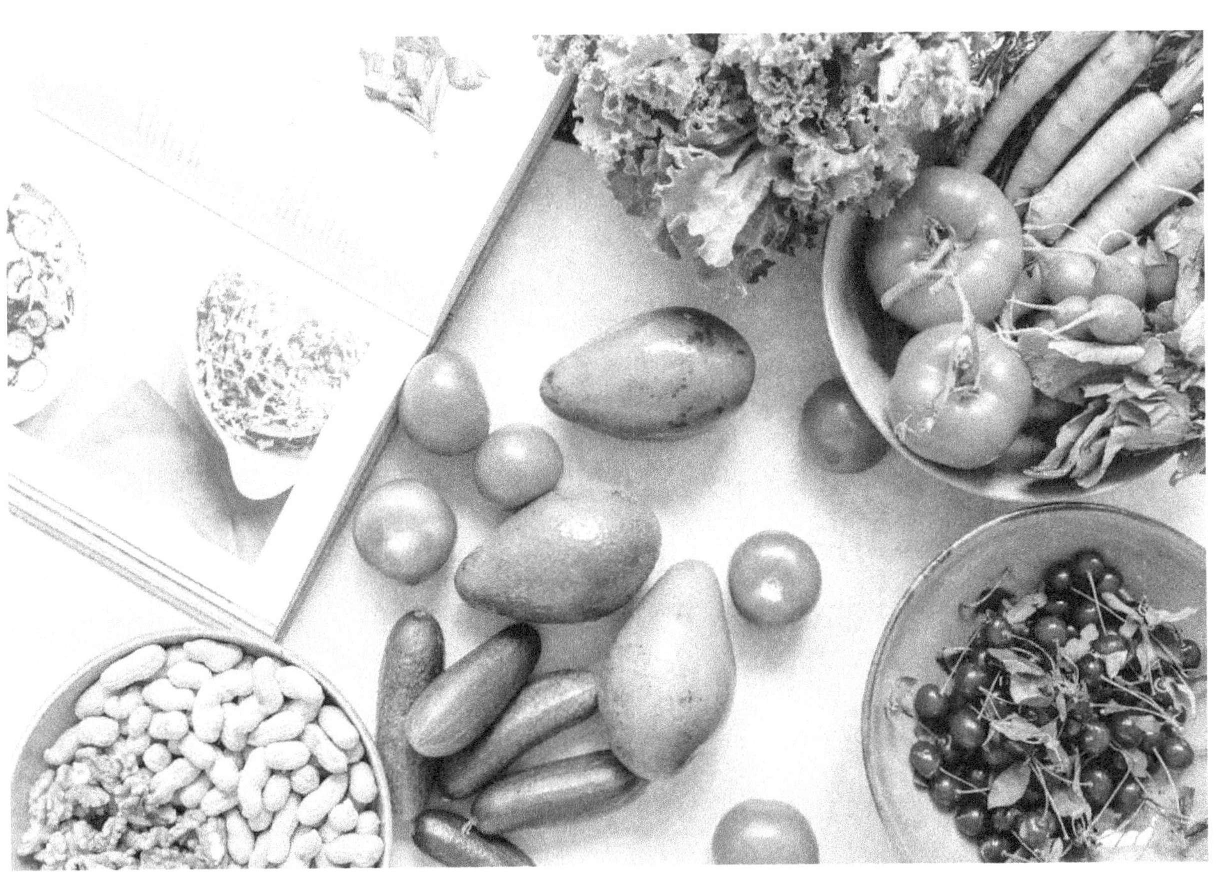

CHAPTER 2

Salad and Side Dishes Recipes

Introduction:

Salads and side dishes play a crucial role in the DASH (Dietary Approaches to Stop Hypertension) diet, as they are typically rich in vegetables, fruits, whole grains, and lean proteins. Here are ten delicious and nutritious salad and side dish recipes designed to help lower blood pressure and promote overall heart health.

1. Spinach and Strawberry Salad

Ingredients:

4 cups baby spinach leaves

1 cup sliced strawberries

1/4 cup sliced almonds

2 tablespoons balsamic vinegar

1 tablespoon olive oil

1 teaspoon honey

Salt and pepper to taste

Instructions:

Combine spinach, almonds, and strawberries in a big bowl.

Combine the olive oil, honey, balsamic vinegar, salt, and pepper in a small bowl.

Over the salad, drizzle with the dressing and toss to coat evenly

Serve immediately.

Nutrients: Rich in antioxidants, fiber, vitamins, and minerals.

Prep Time: 10 minutes.

2. Quinoa Tabouleh

Ingredients:

1 cup cooked quinoa

1 cucumber, diced

1 cup cherry tomatoes, halved

1/4 cup chopped fresh parsley

2 tablespoons lemon juice

1 tablespoon olive oil

Salt and pepper to taste

Instructions:

In a large bowl, combine cooked quinoa, cucumber, tomatoes, and parsley.

In a small bowl, whisk together lemon juice, olive oil, salt, and pepper.

Pour dressing over the quinoa mixture and toss to combine.

Serve chilled or at room temperature.

Nutrients: High in protein, fiber, vitamins, and minerals.

Prep Time: 15 minutes.

3. Greek Cucumber Salad

Ingredients:

2 large cucumbers, sliced

1 cup cherry tomatoes, halved

1/4 cup sliced red onion

1/4 cup crumbled feta cheese

2 tablespoons chopped fresh dill

2 tablespoons lemon juice

1 tablespoon olive oil

Salt and pepper to taste

Instructions:

In a large bowl, combine cucumbers, tomatoes, red onion, feta cheese, and dill.

In a small bowl, whisk together lemon juice, olive oil, salt, and pepper.

Pour dressing over the salad and toss gently to coat.

Serve chilled.

Nutrients: Loaded with hydration, fiber, antioxidants, and healthy fats. **Prep Time:** 10 minutes.

4. Roasted Vegetable Medley

Ingredients:

Two cups of mixed veggies, including carrots, bell peppers, and zucchini

2 tablespoons olive oil

1 teaspoon dried herbs (such as thyme, rosemary, oregano)

Salt and pepper to taste

Instructions:

Preheat oven to 400°F (200°C).

Put the chopped veggies on a baking sheet in bite-sized pieces.

Add a drizzle of olive oil and season with salt, pepper, and dried herbs

Toss to coat evenly.

Roast in the oven for 20-25 minutes, or until vegetables are tender and slightly browned.

Serve hot as a side dish.

Nutrients: Rich in fiber, vitamins, minerals, and antioxidants.

Prep Time: 15 minutes.

5. Caprese Salad

Ingredients:

2 large tomatoes, sliced

1 ball fresh mozzarella cheese, sliced

1/4 cup fresh basil leaves

2 tablespoons balsamic glaze

Salt and pepper to taste

Instructions:

Arrange tomato and mozzarella slices alternately on a serving platter.

Tuck fresh basil leaves between the slices.

Drizzle with balsamic glaze.

Season with salt and pepper to taste.

Serve immediately.

Nutrients: High in calcium, vitamin C, antioxidants, and healthy fats.

Prep Time: 10 minutes.

6. Steamed Asparagus with Lemon

Ingredients:

1 bunch asparagus, trimmed

1 tablespoon olive oil

1 tablespoon lemon juice

Salt and pepper to taste

Instructions:

Steam asparagus in a steamer basket over boiling water for 4-5 minutes, or until tender-crisp.

Transfer steamed asparagus to a serving dish.

Drizzle with olive oil and lemon juice.

Season with salt and pepper to taste.

Serve hot.

Nutrients: Packed with fiber, folate, vitamins, and antioxidants.

Prep Time: 10 minutes.

7. Kale and Apple Salad

Ingredients:

4 cups chopped kale leaves

1 apple, thinly sliced

1/4 cup dried cranberries

1/4 cup chopped walnuts

2 tablespoons apple cider vinegar

1 tablespoon honey

1 tablespoon Dijon mustard

Salt and pepper to taste

Instructions:

In a large bowl, combine kale, apple slices, dried cranberries, and walnuts.

Combine the apple cider vinegar, honey, Dijon mustard, salt, and pepper in a small bowl.

Drizzle the salad with the dressing, tossing to coat thoroughly

Serve immediately.

Nutrients: Rich in fiber, vitamin K, antioxidants, and healthy fats.

Prep Time: 15 minutes.

8. Quinoa and Black Bean Salad

Ingredients:

1 cup cooked quinoa

1 can black beans, drained and rinsed

1 bell pepper, diced

1/4 cup chopped cilantro

2 tablespoons lime juice

1 tablespoon olive oil

1 teaspoon cumin

Salt and pepper to taste

Instructions:

In a large bowl, combine cooked quinoa, black beans, bell pepper, and cilantro.

In a small bowl, whisk together lime juice, olive oil, cumin, salt, and pepper.

Drizzle the salad with the dressing and toss to mix.

Serve chilled or at room temperature.

Nutrients: High in protein, fiber, vitamins, and minerals.

Prep Time: 15 minutes.

9. Edamame and Corn Salad

Ingredients:

1 cup shelled edamame, cooked

1 cup corn kernels, cooked

1/4 cup diced red bell pepper

1/4 cup diced red onion

2 tablespoons chopped fresh cilantro

2 tablespoons lime juice

1 tablespoon olive oil

Salt and pepper to taste

Instructions:

In a large bowl, combine cooked edamame, corn, bell pepper, onion, and cilantro.

In a small bowl, whisk together lime juice, olive oil, salt, and pepper.

Drizzle the salad with the dressing, tossing to coat thoroughly

Serve chilled.

Nutrients: Rich in protein, fiber, antioxidants, and vitamins.

Prep Time: 10 minutes.

10. Roasted Sweet Potato Wedges

Ingredients:

2 large sweet potatoes, cut into wedges

2 tablespoons olive oil

1 teaspoon paprika

1 teaspoon garlic powder

Salt and pepper to taste

Instructions:

Preheat oven to 400°F (200°C).

In a large bowl, toss sweet potato wedges with olive oil, paprika, garlic powder, salt, and pepper until evenly coated.

Place the wedges on a baking sheet in a single layer.

Roast in the oven for 25-30 minutes, flipping halfway through, until tender and golden brown.

Serve hot as a side dish.

Nutrients: High in fiber, vitamins A and C, potassium, and antioxidants.

Prep Time: 10 minutes.

CHAPTER 3

Fish and Seafood Recipes

Introduction:

The DASH (Dietary Approaches to Stop Hypertension) diet emphasizes consuming foods that are rich in nutrients like potassium, calcium, and magnesium, which are known to lower blood pressure. Fish and seafood are excellent choices for DASH diet recipes as they are high in omega-3 fatty acids, which promote heart health. Here are 10 healthy DASH diet fish and seafood recipes to support lower blood pressure and overall heart health.

1. Grilled Salmon with Lemon and Herbs

Ingredients:

Salmon fillets

Fresh lemon

Fresh herbs, such thyme, parsley, or dill

Olive oil

Salt and pepper

Instructions:

Preheat grill to medium-high heat.

Brush salmon fillets with olive oil and season with salt, pepper, and chopped herbs.

Grill salmon for about 4-5 minutes per side until cooked through.

Before serving, squeeze some fresh lemon juice over the salmon.

Nutrients: High in omega-3 fatty acids, protein, and vitamin D.

Prep Time: 15 minutes

2. Baked Cod with Tomato and Basil

Ingredients:

Cod fillets

Fresh tomatoes

Fresh basil

Garlic cloves

Olive oil

Salt and pepper

Instructions:

Preheat oven to 375°F (190°C).

Place cod fillets in a baking dish.

Chop tomatoes, basil, and garlic, then mix with olive oil, salt, and pepper.

Spread tomato mixture over the cod fillets.

Bake for 15-20 minutes until fish is cooked through.

Nutrients: Abundant in vitamins, antioxidants, and omega-3 fatty acids.

Prep Time: 20 minutes

3. Shrimp and Vegetable Stir-Fry

Ingredients:

Shrimp

Vegetable mixtures (including broccoli, snap peas, and bell peppers)

Garlic

Ginger

Soy sauce

Olive oil

Instructions:

In a skillet set over medium-high heat, warm the olive oil.

Add minced garlic and ginger, then stir in shrimp.

Cook until shrimp turns pink, then add mixed vegetables and soy sauce.

Stir-fry until vegetables are tender-crisp.

Serve hot.

Nutrients: Low in calories, high in protein, and fiber.

Prep Time: 20 minutes

4. Tuna Salad with Avocado

Ingredients:

Canned tuna

Ripe avocado

Red onion

Celery

Lemon juice

Dijon mustard

Salt and pepper

Instructions:

Place the drained canned tuna in a bowl.

Mash avocado and mix with tuna.

Add chopped red onion, celery, lemon juice, Dijon mustard, salt, and pepper.

Stir until well combined.

Serve on whole-grain bread or lettuce leaves.

Nutrients: High in omega-3 fatty acids, fiber, and potassium.

Prep Time: 10 minutes

5. Lemon Garlic Grilled Shrimp Skewers

Ingredients:

Shrimp

Fresh lemon juice

Garlic cloves

Olive oil

Salt and pepper

Instructions:

In a bowl, mix lemon juice, minced garlic, olive oil, salt, and pepper.

For fifteen minutes, marinate the shrimp in the marinade.

Thread shrimp onto skewers.

Grill skewers over medium-high heat for 2-3 minutes per side.

Serve hot with lemon wedges.

Nutrients: Low in calories, high in protein, and vitamin C.

Prep Time: 20 minutes

6. Seared Scallops with Mango Salsa

Ingredients:

Scallops

Ripe mango

Red bell pepper

Red onion

Cilantro

Lime juice

Olive oil

Salt and pepper

Instructions:

After patting dry, season scallops with salt & pepper.

In a skillet over high heat, warm the olive oil.

Sear scallops till golden brown, 2 to 3 minutes per side

Dice mango, bell pepper, and red onion, then mix with chopped cilantro, lime juice, salt, and pepper to make salsa.

Serve seared scallops with mango salsa on top.

Nutrients: High in protein, antioxidants, and vitamin C.

Prep Time: 20 minutes

7. Grilled Swordfish with Mediterranean Salsa

Ingredients:

Swordfish steaks

Cherry tomatoes

Kalamata olives

Cucumber

Red onion

Fresh parsley

Olive oil

Balsamic vinegar

Salt and pepper

Instructions:

Season swordfish steaks with salt, pepper, and olive oil.

Grill swordfish over medium-high heat for 4-5 minutes per side until cooked through.

Dice tomatoes, olives, cucumber, red onion, and parsley to make salsa.

Toss salsa ingredients with olive oil, balsamic vinegar, salt, and pepper.

Serve grilled swordfish topped with Mediterranean salsa.

Nutrients: Abundant in vitamins, antioxidants, and omega-3 fatty acids.

Prep Time: 25 minutes

8. Baked Halibut with Pesto Crust

Ingredients:

Halibut fillets

Pesto sauce

Breadcrumbs

Olive oil

Salt and pepper

Instructions:

Preheat oven to 400°F (200°C).

Place halibut fillets on a baking dish.

Spread pesto sauce over the top of each fillet.

Sprinkle breadcrumbs on top of the pesto.

Drizzle olive oil over the breadcrumbs and season with salt and pepper.

Bake for 15-20 minutes until fish is cooked through and topping is golden brown.

Nutrients: High in protein, omega-3 fatty acids, and antioxidants.

Prep Time: 25 minutes

9. Salmon and Quinoa Salad

Ingredients:

Cooked salmon flakes

Cooked quinoa

Cherry tomatoes

Cucumber

Red onion

Feta cheese

Fresh dill

Lemon vinaigrette dressing

Instructions:

In a large bowl, combine cooked salmon flakes, cooked quinoa, halved cherry tomatoes, diced cucumber, thinly sliced red onion, crumbled feta cheese, and chopped fresh dill.

Toss with lemon vinaigrette dressing until evenly coated.

Serve chilled or at room temperature.

Nutrients: High in protein, fiber, omega-3 fatty acids, and vitamins.

Prep Time: 25 minutes

10. Tuna Stuffed Bell Peppers

Ingredients:

Bell peppers

Canned tuna

Cooked brown rice

Black beans

Corn kernels

Salsa

Shredded cheddar cheese

Fresh cilantro

Instructions:

Preheat oven to 375°F (190°C).

Remove the seeds and membranes from the bell peppers by cutting off the tops

In a bowl, mix canned tuna, cooked brown rice, black beans, corn kernels, and salsa.

Stuff each bell pepper with the tuna mixture.

Top stuffed peppers with shredded cheddar cheese and arrange in a baking dish.

Bake the peppers for 25 to 30 minutes with a foil cover until they are soft

Garnish with fresh cilantro before serving.

Nutrients: Rich in vitamins, minerals, fiber, and protein.

Prep Time: 30 minutes

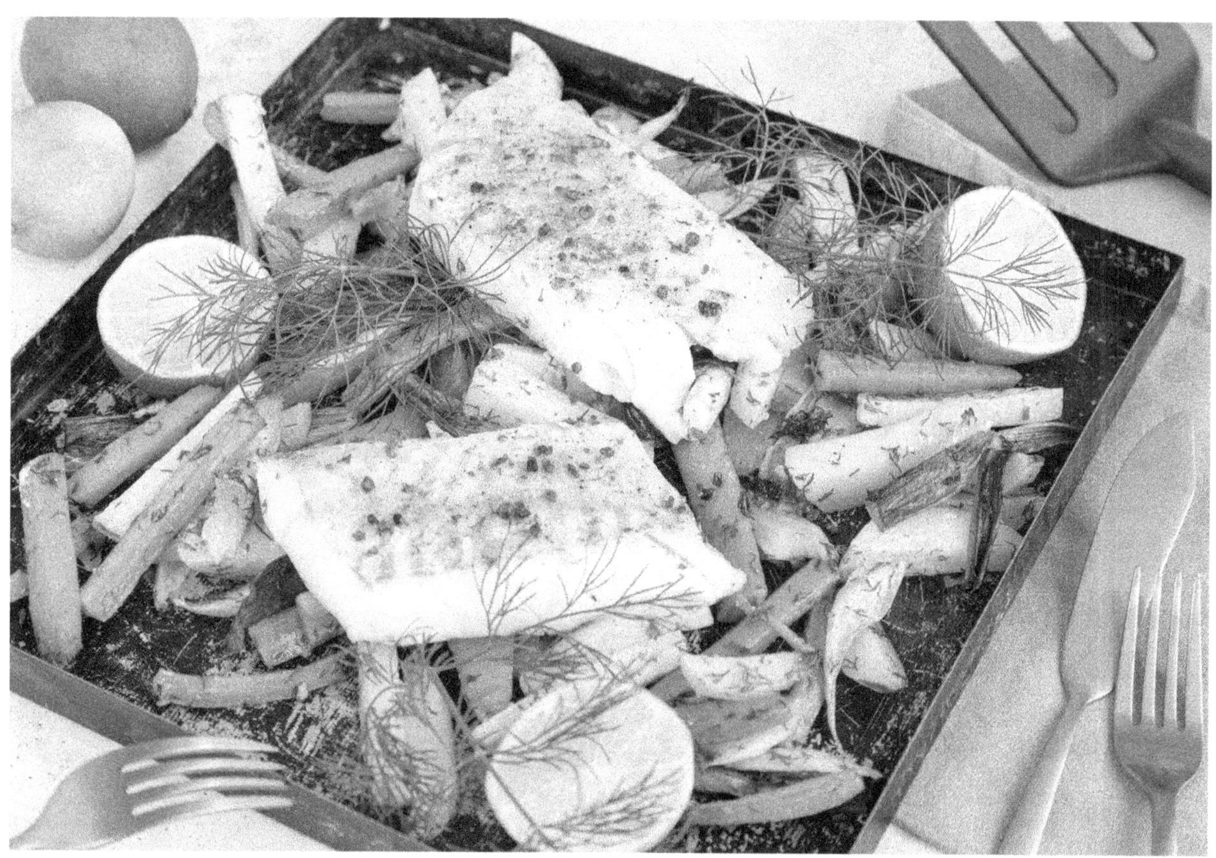

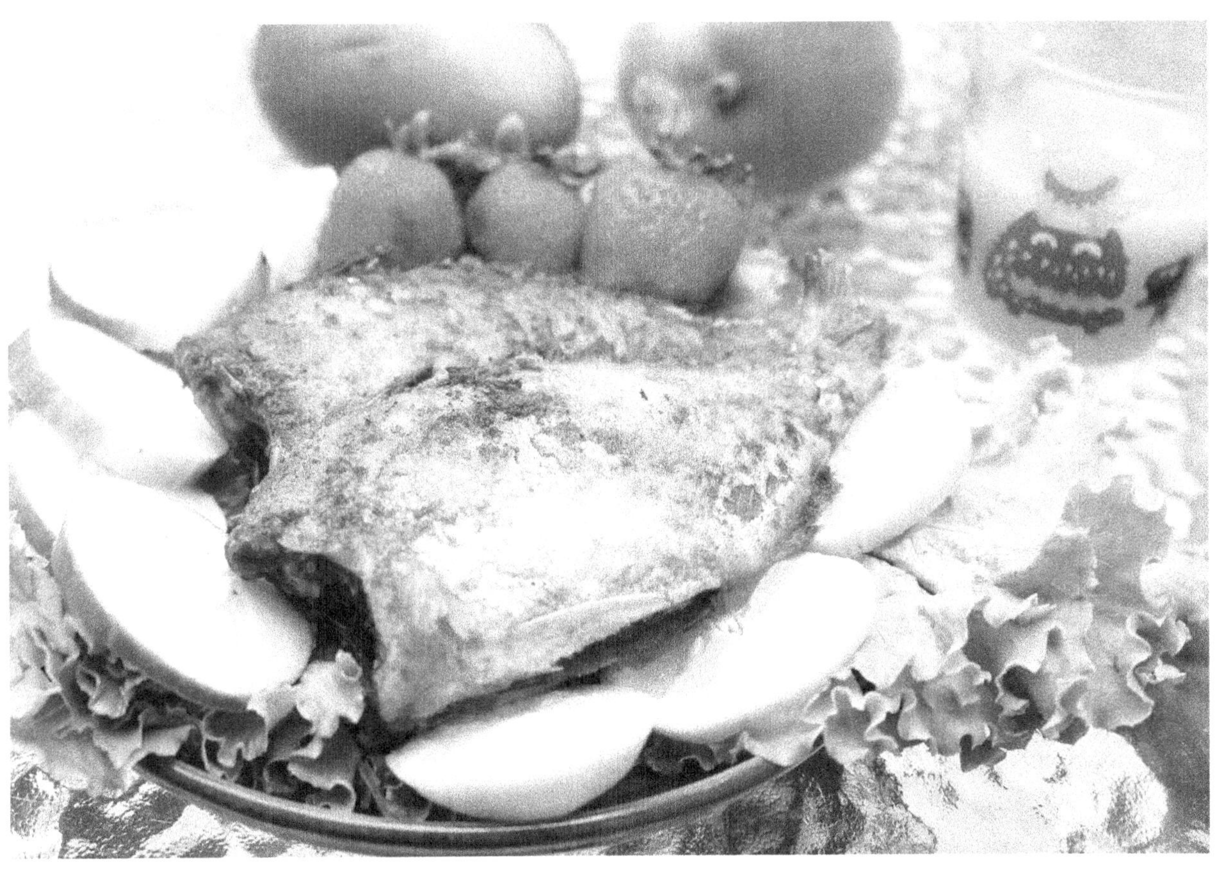

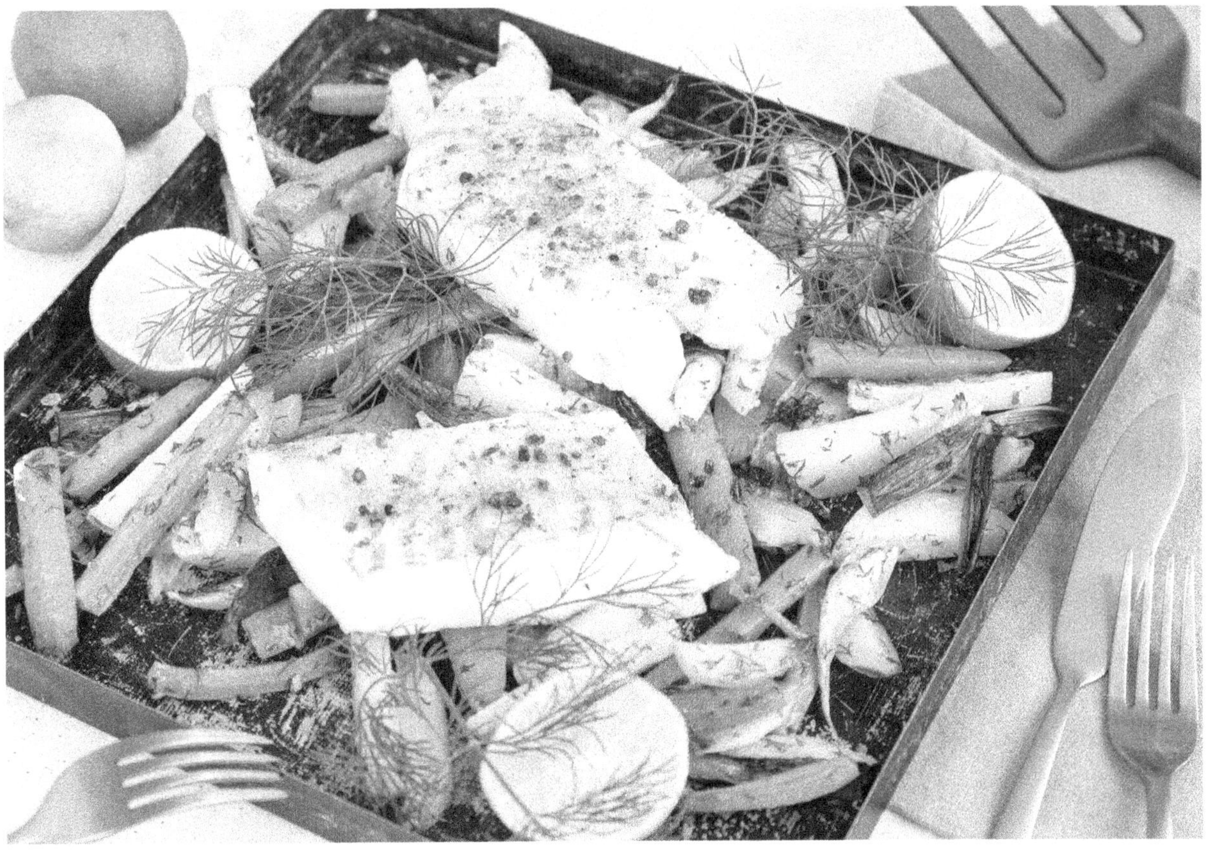

CHAPTER 4

Grain and Bean Recipes

Introduction:

The DASH (Dietary Approaches to Stop Hypertension) diet emphasizes foods that are rich in nutrients like potassium, calcium, and magnesium, which are known to lower blood pressure. Incorporating grains and beans into your diet can provide fiber, protein, and essential vitamins and minerals that support heart health. Here are 10 healthy DASH diet grain and bean recipes to help lower blood pressure and promote overall heart health.

1. Quinoa and Black Bean Salad

Ingredients:

Quinoa

Black beans

Bell peppers

Red onion

Cilantro

Lime juice

Olive oil

Salt and pepper

Instructions:

As directed on the package, prepare the quinoa and allow it to cool

Rinse and drain black beans.

Dice bell peppers and red onion, and chop cilantro.

In a bowl, combine cooked quinoa, black beans, bell peppers, red onion, and cilantro.

Dress with lime juice, olive oil, salt, and pepper.

Toss until well combined.

Serve chilled or at room temperature.

Nutrients: High in fiber, protein, antioxidants, and vitamins.

Prep Time: 20 minutes

2. Lentil Vegetable Soup

Ingredients:

Lentils

Carrots

Celery

Onion

Garlic

Vegetable broth

Bay leaves

Thyme

Salt and pepper

Instructions:

Rinse lentils and set aside.

Chop carrots, celery, onion, and garlic.

In a pot, sauté onion and garlic until fragrant.

Add carrots and celery, and cook until slightly softened.

Pour in vegetable broth, add lentils, bay leaves, and thyme.

Simmer for about 25-30 minutes until lentils are tender.

Season with salt and pepper to taste.

Serve hot.

Nutrients: High in fiber, protein, vitamins, and minerals.

Prep Time: 30 minutes

3. Brown Rice and Vegetable Stir-Fry

Ingredients:

Brown rice

Vegetable mixtures (including snap peas, broccoli, and bell peppers)

Garlic

Ginger

Soy sauce

Olive oil

Instructions:

Cook brown rice according to package instructions and set aside.

In a skillet set over medium-high heat, warm the olive oil.

Add minced garlic and ginger, then stir in mixed vegetables.

Cook until vegetables are tender-crisp.

Add cooked brown rice and soy sauce to the skillet.

Stir-fry until well combined.

Serve hot.

Nutrients: High in fiber, antioxidants, and vitamins.

Prep Time: 25 minutes

4. Chickpea and Spinach Curry

Ingredients:

Chickpeas

Spinach

Onion

Garlic

Tomato sauce

Coconut milk

Curry powder

Turmeric

Cumin

Salt and pepper

Instructions:

In a pot, sauté minced garlic and chopped onion until softened

Add curry powder, turmeric, and cumin, and cook until fragrant.

Pour in tomato sauce and coconut milk.

After adding the drained chickpeas, simmer

Stir in spinach and cook until wilted.

Season with salt and pepper to taste.

Serve hot over cooked rice or quinoa.

Nutrients: High in fiber, protein, antioxidants, and iron.

Prep Time: 30 minutes

5. Whole Wheat Pasta Primavera

Ingredients:

Whole wheat pasta

Mixed vegetables, including bell peppers, cherry tomatoes, and zucchini

Garlic

Olive oil

Fresh basil

Parmesan cheese (optional)

Salt and pepper

Instructions:

Cook whole wheat pasta according to package instructions and set aside.

In a skillet over medium heat, warm the olive oil.

Sauté minced garlic until fragrant.

Add mixed vegetables and cook until tender.

Toss cooked pasta with vegetables in the skillet.

Season with salt and pepper.

Serve hot, garnished with fresh basil and Parmesan cheese if desired.

Nutrients: High in fiber, antioxidants, vitamins, and minerals.

Prep Time: 25 minutes

6. Black Bean and Sweet Potato Tacos

Ingredients:

Black beans

Sweet potatoes

Onion

Garlic

Cumin

Chili powder

Tortillas

Avocado

Cilantro

Lime wedges

Instructions:

Roast diced sweet potatoes in the oven until tender.

Sauté chopped onion and minced garlic in a skillet until softened.

Add drained black beans, cumin, and chili powder to the skillet.

Cook until flavors are blended and food is thoroughly heated

Warm tortillas and fill with black bean mixture and roasted sweet potatoes.

Top with sliced avocado and chopped cilantro.

Serve with lime wedges.

Nutrients: High in fiber, protein, antioxidants, and vitamins.

Prep Time: 30 minutes

7. Quinoa Stuffed Bell Peppers

Ingredients:

Quinoa

Bell peppers

Black beans

Corn kernels

Onion

Garlic

Tomato sauce

Cumin

Paprika

Salt and pepper

Instructions:

Prepare the quinoa as directed on the package and reserve.

Remove the seeds and membranes from bell peppers by cutting off the tops

Sauté chopped onion and minced garlic in a skillet until softened.

Stir in cooked quinoa, black beans, corn kernels, tomato sauce, cumin, paprika, salt, and pepper.

Spoon quinoa mixture into bell peppers.

Bake stuffed peppers in the oven at 375°F (190°C) for 25-30 minutes until peppers are tender.

Serve hot.

Nutrients: High in fiber, protein, antioxidants, and vitamins.

Prep Time: 35 minutes

8. Barley and Vegetable Soup

Ingredients:

Barley

Carrots

Celery

Onion

Garlic

Vegetable broth

Thyme

Bay leaves

Salt and pepper

Instructions:

Rinse barley and set aside.

Chop carrots, celery, onion, and garlic.

In a pot, sauté onion and garlic until fragrant.

Add carrots and celery, and cook until slightly softened.

Pour in vegetable broth, add barley, bay leaves, and thyme.

Simmer for about 30-35 minutes until barley is tender.

Season with salt and pepper to taste.

Serve hot.

Nutrients: High in fiber, protein, antioxidants, and minerals.

Prep Time: 40 minutes

9. Chickpea and Quinoa Salad

Ingredients:

Chickpeas

Quinoa

Cucumber

Cherry tomatoes

Red onion

Parsley

Lemon juice

Olive oil

Instructions:

As directed on the package, prepare the quinoa and allow it to cool

Rinse and drain chickpeas.

Dice cucumber, halve cherry tomatoes, and finely chop red onion and parsley.

In a large bowl, combine cooked quinoa, chickpeas, cucumber, cherry tomatoes, red onion, and parsley.

Add some olive oil and lemon juice to the salad.

Toss until well combined.

Serve chilled or at room temperature.

Nutrients: High in fiber, protein, antioxidants, and vitamins.

Prep Time: 25 minutes

10. Brown Rice and Black Bean Burrito Bowl

Ingredients:

Brown rice

Black beans

Avocado

Tomato salsa

Corn kernels

Red onion

Cilantro

Lime wedges

Instructions:

Cook brown rice according to package instructions and set aside.

Rinse and drain black beans.

Dice avocado and finely chop red onion and cilantro.

In serving bowls, layer cooked brown rice, black beans, avocado, tomato salsa, corn kernels, red onion, and cilantro.

Before serving, squeeze some lime wedges over the bowl.

Serve hot or at room temperature.

Nutrients: High in fiber, protein, antioxidants, and healthy fats.

Prep Time: 30 minutes

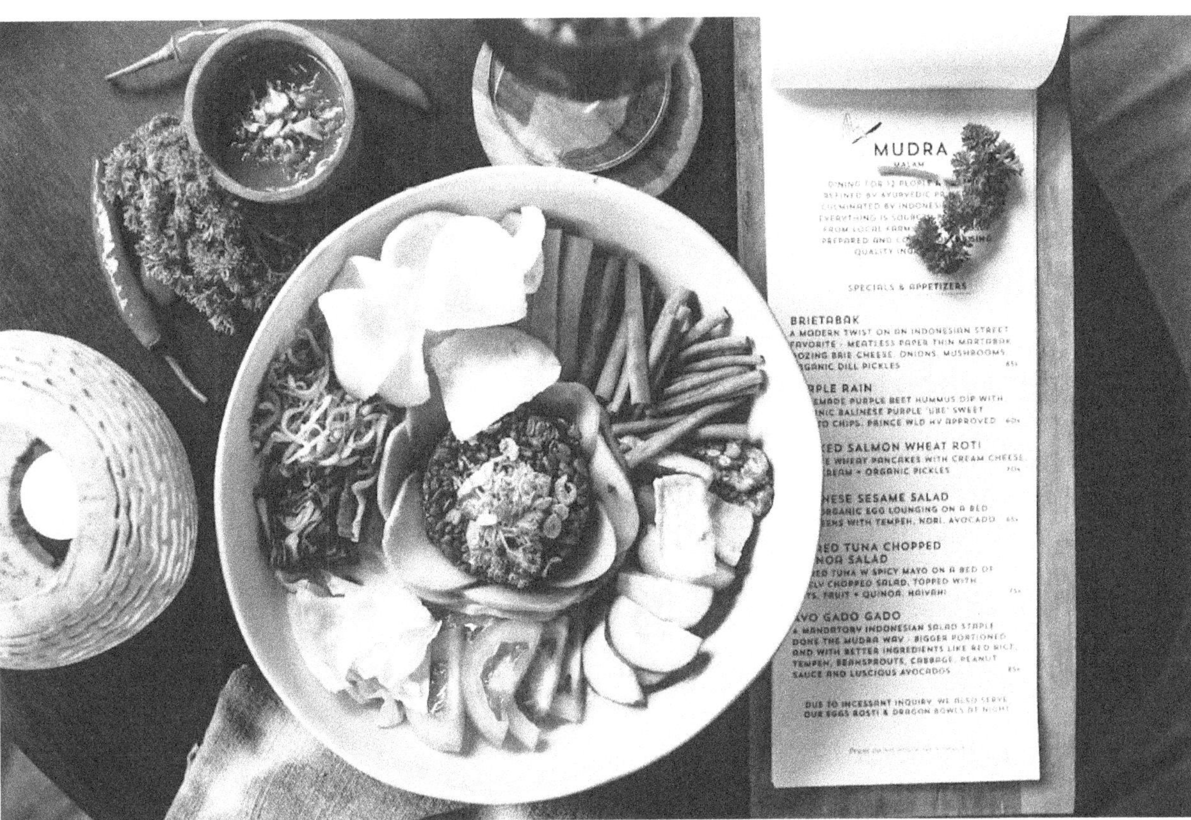
MUDRA
MALAM

DINING FOR 12 PEOPLE
REFINED BY AYURVEDIC PR
CULMINATED BY INDONESI
EVERYTHING IS SOURCE
FROM LOCAL FARM
PREPARED AND C
QUALITY ING

SPECIALS & APPETIZERS

BRIETABAK
A MODERN TWIST ON AN INDONESIAN STREET
FAVORITE - MEATLESS PAPER THIN MARTABAK
OOZING BRIE CHEESE, ONIONS, MUSHROOMS
ORGANIC DILL PICKLES   65.

PURPLE RAIN
HOMEMADE PURPLE BEET HUMMUS DIP WITH
ICONIC BALINESE PURPLE 'UBE' SWEET
POTATO CHIPS, PRINCE WLD HV APPROVED   60.

SMOKED SALMON WHEAT ROTI
WHEAT PANCAKES WITH CREAM CHEESE
CREAM + ORGANIC PICKLES   70.

BALINESE SESAME SALAD
ORGANIC EGG LOUNGING ON A BED
OF GREENS WITH TEMPEH, NORI, AVOCADO   65.

SEARED TUNA CHOPPED
QUINOA SALAD
SEARED TUNA W SPICY MAYO ON A BED OF
FINELY CHOPPED SALAD, TOPPED WITH
NUTS, FRUIT + QUINOA, HAIVAH!   75.

AVO GADO GADO
A MANDATORY INDONESIAN SALAD STAPLE
DONE THE MUDRA WAY - BIGGER PORTIONED
AND WITH BETTER INGREDIENTS LIKE RED RICE,
TEMPEH, BEANSPROUTS, CABBAGE, PEANUT
SAUCE AND LUSCIOUS AVOCADOS   85.

DUE TO INCESSANT INQUIRY, WE ALSO SERVE
OUR EGGS ROSTI & DRAGON BOWLS AT NIGHT

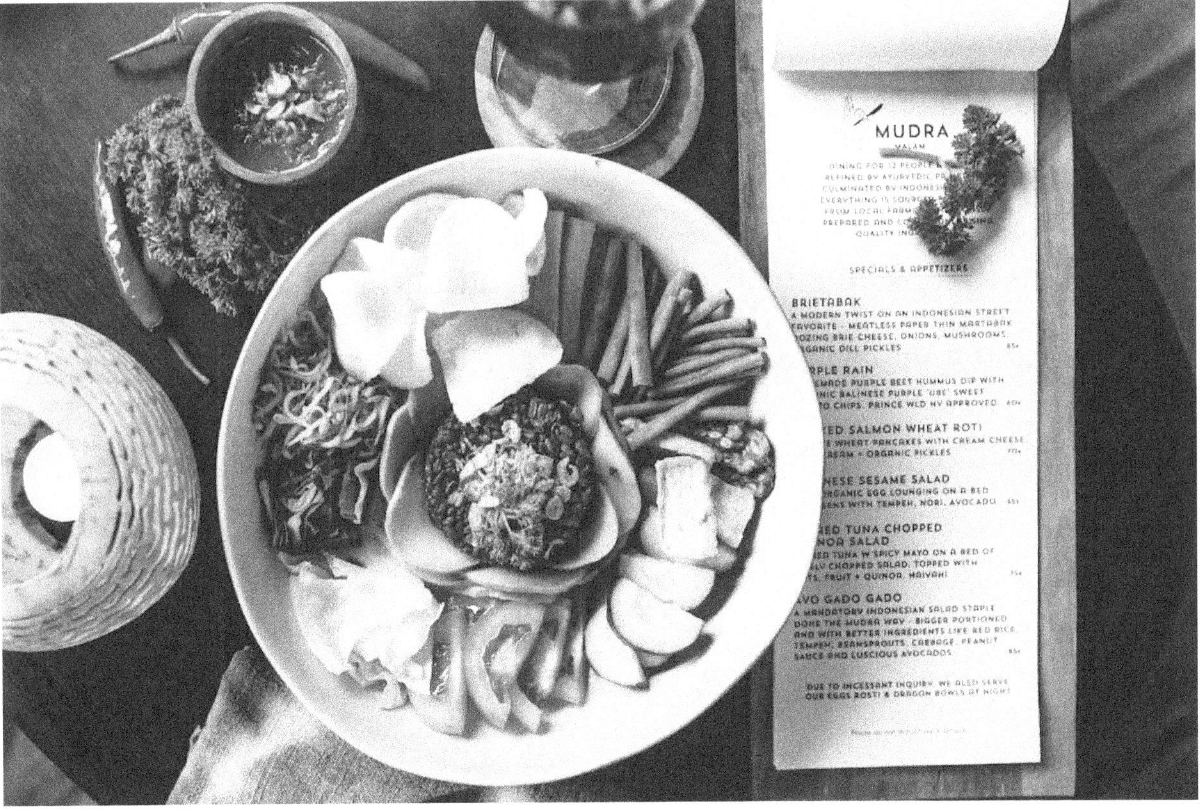
MUDRA
MALAM

DINING FOR 12 PEOPLE
REFINED BY AYURVEDIC PR
CULMINATED BY INDONESI
EVERYTHING IS SOURCE
FROM LOCAL FARM
PREPARED AND C
QUALITY IN

SPECIALS & APPETIZERS

BRIETABAK
A MODERN TWIST ON AN INDONESIAN STREET
FAVORITE - MEATLESS PAPER THIN MARTABAK
OOZING BRIE CHEESE, ONIONS, MUSHROOMS
ORGANIC DILL PICKLES   65.

PURPLE RAIN
HOMEMADE PURPLE BEET HUMMUS DIP WITH
ICONIC BALINESE PURPLE 'UBE' SWEET
POTATO CHIPS, PRINCE WLD HV APPROVED   60.

SMOKED SALMON WHEAT ROTI
WHEAT PANCAKES WITH CREAM CHEESE
CREAM + ORGANIC PICKLES   70.

BALINESE SESAME SALAD
ORGANIC EGG LOUNGING ON A BED
OF GREENS WITH TEMPEH, NORI, AVOCADO   65.

SEARED TUNA CHOPPED
QUINOA SALAD
SEARED TUNA W SPICY MAYO ON A BED OF
FINELY CHOPPED SALAD, TOPPED WITH
NUTS, FRUIT + QUINOA, HAIVAH!   75.

AVO GADO GADO
A MANDATORY INDONESIAN SALAD STAPLE
DONE THE MUDRA WAY - BIGGER PORTIONED
AND WITH BETTER INGREDIENTS LIKE RED RICE,
TEMPEH, BEANSPROUTS, CABBAGE, PEANUT
SAUCE AND LUSCIOUS AVOCADOS   85.

DUE TO INCESSANT INQUIRY, WE ALSO SERVE
OUR EGGS ROSTI & DRAGON BOWLS AT NIGHT

CHAPTER 5

Vegetarian Recipes

Introduction:

Dietary Approaches to Stop Hypertension, or DASH, is well known for its capacity to reduce blood pressure and strengthen the heart. Emphasizing fruits, vegetables, whole grains, and lean proteins, it's an excellent choice for vegetarians seeking to maintain a healthy lifestyle. Here are 10 delicious vegetarian recipes inspired by the DASH diet, designed to nourish your body and support cardiovascular wellness.

Quinoa-Stuffed Bell Peppers:

Ingredients: Quinoa, bell peppers, black beans, corn, tomatoes, onion, garlic, spices.

Instructions: Cook quinoa. Sauté onion and garlic, then mix with quinoa, beans, corn, and tomatoes. Stuff peppers, bake until tender.

Nutrients: High in fiber, protein, and antioxidants. Low in sodium and saturated fat.

Prep Time: 30 minutes.

Vegetable Stir-Fry with Tofu:

Ingredients: Tofu, mixed vegetables (broccoli, bell peppers, carrots, snap peas), soy sauce, ginger, garlic.

Instructions: Press tofu, stir-fry with vegetables, ginger, and garlic in soy sauce.

Nutrients: Rich in protein, vitamins, and minerals. Low in sodium and saturated fat.

Prep Time: 25 minutes.

Mediterranean Chickpea Salad:

Ingredients: Chickpeas, cucumber, cherry tomatoes, red onion, olives, feta cheese (optional), olive oil, lemon juice, herbs.

Instructions: Mix chickpeas, chopped vegetables, and dressing. Top with feta and herbs.

Nutrients: High in fiber, protein, and healthy fats. Low in sodium.

Prep Time: 15 minutes.

Spinach and Feta Stuffed Portobello Mushrooms:

Ingredients: Portobello mushrooms, spinach, feta cheese, garlic, breadcrumbs.

Instructions: Sauté spinach and garlic, mix with feta and breadcrumbs. Stuff mushrooms, bake until tender.

Nutrients: Rich in iron, calcium, and antioxidants. Low in sodium.

Prep Time: 35 minutes.

Lentil and Vegetable Soup:

Ingredients: Lentils, carrots, celery, onion, garlic, vegetable broth, spices.

Instructions: Sauté vegetables, add lentils, broth, and spices. Simmer until lentils are tender.

Nutrients: High in fiber, protein, and vitamins. Low in sodium and fat.

Prep Time: 40 minutes.

Vegetable and Bean Chili:

Ingredients: Mixed beans (kidney, black beans, pinto beans), tomatoes, bell peppers, onion, garlic, chili powder, cumin.

Instructions: Sauté vegetables, add beans, tomatoes, and spices. Simmer until flavors meld.

Nutrients: Packed with fiber, protein, and antioxidants. Low in sodium and saturated fat.

Prep Time: 45 minutes.

Greek Yogurt and Berry Parfait:

Ingredients: Greek yogurt, mixed berries, honey, granola.

Instructions: Layer yogurt, berries, honey, and granola in a glass.

Nutrients: High in protein, calcium, and antioxidants. Low in sodium and saturated fat.

Prep Time: 10 minutes.

Whole Wheat Veggie Pizza:

Ingredients: Whole wheat pizza dough, tomato sauce, bell peppers, mushrooms, spinach, olives, mozzarella cheese.

Instructions: Roll out dough, spread sauce, top with vegetables and cheese. Bake until crust is golden.

Nutrients: Rich in fiber, vitamins, and minerals. Moderate in sodium and fat.

Prep Time: 30 minutes.

Tofu and Vegetable Kabobs:

Ingredients: Tofu, bell peppers, zucchini, cherry tomatoes, onion, marinade (olive oil, lemon juice, herbs).

Instructions: Cube tofu and vegetables, marinate, thread onto skewers. Grill until tender.

Nutrients: High in protein, vitamins, and antioxidants. Low in sodium and saturated fat.

Prep Time: 35 minutes.

Oatmeal with Mixed Berries and Almonds:

Ingredients: Almond milk, honey, rolled oats, and mixed berries.

Instructions: Cook oats with almond milk, top with berries, almonds, and honey.

Nutrients: High in fiber, protein, and antioxidants. Low in sodium and saturated fat.

Prep Time: 15 minutes.

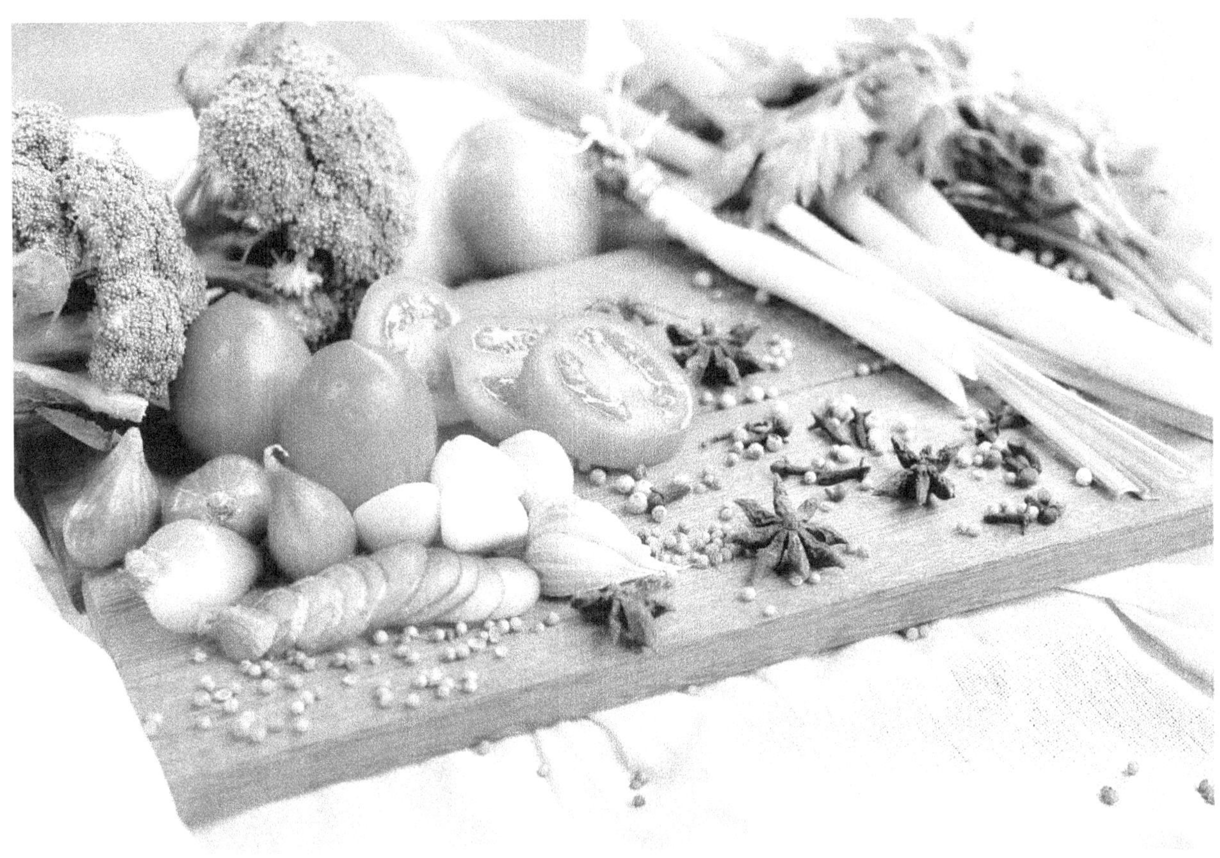

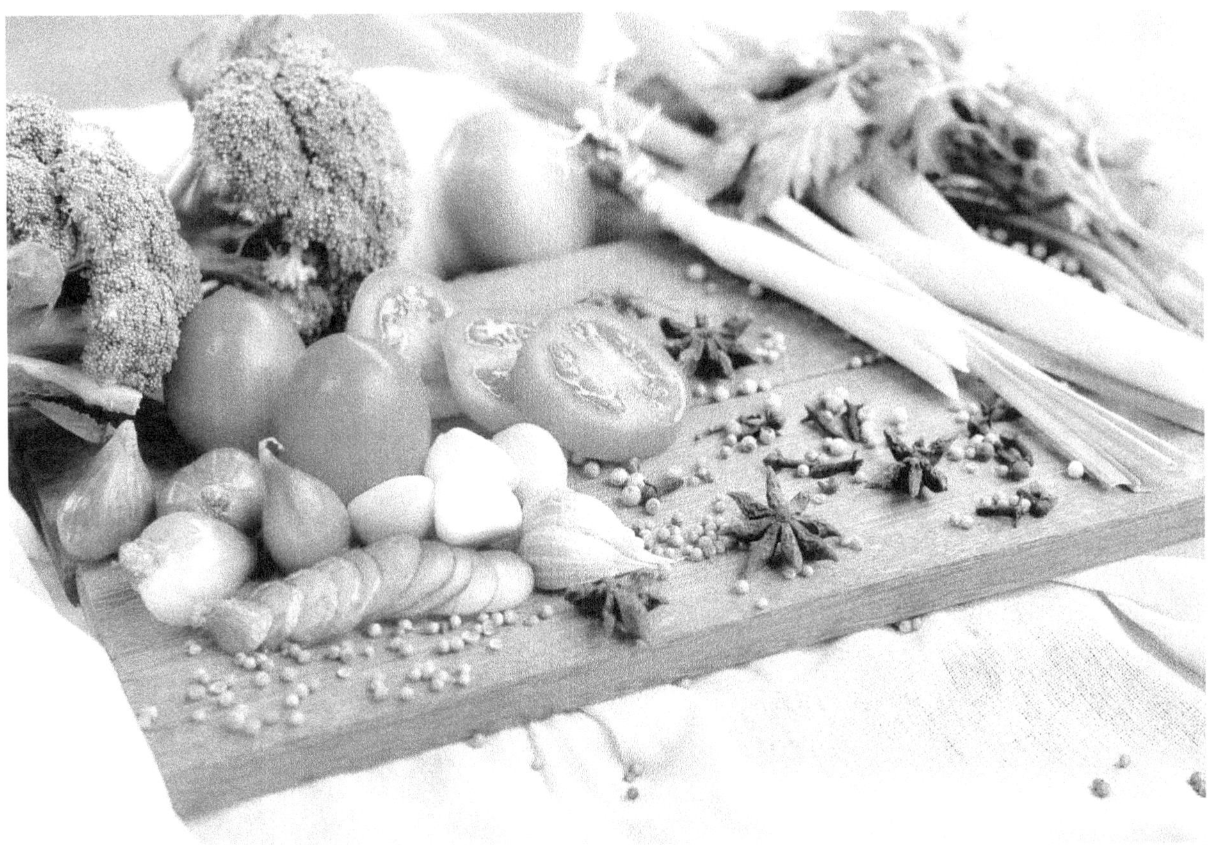

CHAPTER 6

Vegan Recipes

Introduction:

The DASH (Dietary Approaches to Stop Hypertension) diet emphasizes the consumption of nutrient-rich foods to lower blood pressure and promote heart health. Following a vegan version of the DASH diet can provide numerous health benefits, including reduced risk of heart disease and improved overall well-being. Below are 10 delicious and nutritious vegan recipes that align with the principles of the DASH diet.

1. Quinoa Vegetable Stir-Fry

Ingredients:

1 cup quinoa

a variety of veggies, including snap peas, broccoli, carrots, and bell peppers

2 cloves garlic, minced

1 tablespoon olive oil

Low-sodium soy sauce

1 teaspoon ginger, grated

Instructions:

Cook quinoa according to package instructions.

In a large skillet, heat olive oil over medium heat. Add the ginger and garlic, and cook until aromatic.

Add assorted vegetables and stir-fry until tender.

Stir in cooked quinoa and soy sauce, cook for an additional 2-3 minutes.

Serve hot.

Nutrients: High in fiber, protein, vitamins, and minerals. Low in sodium and saturated fat.

Prep Time: 25 minutes

2. Lentil and Vegetable Soup

Ingredients:

1 cup lentils, rinsed

Assorted vegetables (carrots, celery, tomatoes, spinach)

4 cups vegetable broth

2 cloves garlic, minced

1 teaspoon dried thyme

Salt and pepper to taste

Instructions:

Garlic should be softened and aromatic in a big pot.

Add lentils, assorted vegetables, thyme, and vegetable broth. Bring to a boil.

Reduce heat and simmer until lentils are tender, about 25-30 minutes.

Season with salt and pepper to taste.

Serve hot.

Nutrients: High in fiber, protein, vitamins, and minerals. Low in sodium and saturated fat.

Prep Time: 35 minutes

3. Chickpea and Vegetable Curry

Ingredients:

1 can chickpeas, drained and rinsed

Assorted vegetables (bell peppers, cauliflower, peas)

1 can coconut milk

2 tablespoons curry powder

2 cloves garlic, minced

1 tablespoon olive oil

Instructions:

In a large skillet, heat olive oil over medium heat. Add garlic and sauté until fragrant.

Add assorted vegetables and chickpeas, cook until tender.

Stir in curry powder and coconut milk. Simmer for 10-15 minutes.

Serve hot with rice or quinoa.

Nutrients: Rich in protein, fiber, and essential nutrients. Low in sodium and saturated fat.

Prep Time: 30 minutes

4. Spinach and Mushroom Stuffed Bell Peppers

Ingredients:

4 bell peppers

2 cups spinach, chopped

1 cup mushrooms, diced

1 cup cooked quinoa

1/2 cup tomato sauce

1 teaspoon Italian seasoning

Salt and pepper to taste

Instructions:

Preheat oven to 375°F (190°C).

Remove seeds and cut the tops off the bell peppers.

In a skillet, sauté mushrooms until tender. Add spinach and cook until wilted.

Stir in cooked quinoa, tomato sauce, Italian seasoning, salt, and pepper.

Stuff bell peppers with the quinoa mixture.

Bake peppers for 25 to 30 minutes, or until soft.

Serve hot.

Nutrients: High in fiber, vitamins, and minerals. Low in sodium and saturated fat.

Prep Time: 45 minutes

5. Black Bean and Corn Salad

Ingredients:

1 can black beans, drained and rinsed

1 cup corn kernels

1 bell pepper, diced

1/4 cup red onion, finely chopped

1/4 cup cilantro, chopped

Juice of 1 lime

1 tablespoon olive oil

Salt and pepper to taste

Instructions:

In a large bowl, combine black beans, corn, bell pepper, red onion, and cilantro.

In a small bowl, whisk together lime juice, olive oil, salt, and pepper.

Drizzle the salad with the dressing and toss to coat.

Serve chilled or at room temperature.

Nutrients: Rich in fiber, protein, vitamins, and minerals. Low in sodium and saturated fat.

Prep Time: 15 minutes

6. Mediterranean Quinoa Salad

Ingredients:

1 cup quinoa

1 cucumber, diced

1 cup cherry tomatoes, halved

1/4 cup Kalamata olives, sliced

1/4 cup red onion, finely chopped

1/4 cup fresh parsley, chopped

Juice of 1 lemon

2 tablespoons olive oil

Salt and pepper to taste

Instructions:

Cook quinoa according to package instructions.

In a large bowl, combine cooked quinoa, cucumber, tomatoes, olives, red onion, and parsley.

In a small bowl, whisk together lemon juice, olive oil, salt, and pepper.

Drizzle salad with dressing, tossing to coat.

Serve chilled or at room temperature.

Nutrients: High in fiber, protein, vitamins, and minerals. Low in sodium and saturated fat.

Prep Time: 20 minutes

7. Tofu and Vegetable Stir-Fry

Ingredients:

1 block tofu, pressed and cubed

Assorted vegetables (broccoli, bell peppers, carrots)

2 cloves garlic, minced

2 tablespoons soy sauce

1 tablespoon maple syrup

1 tablespoon sesame oil

Instructions:

Sesame oil should be heated over medium heat in a big skillet

Add garlic and sauté until fragrant.

Tofu cubes should be added and cooked until golden brown all over

Add assorted vegetables and stir-fry until tender.

In a small bowl, whisk together soy sauce and maple syrup. Pour over tofu and vegetables.

Cook for an additional 2-3 minutes, until sauce thickens.

Serve hot with rice or quinoa.

Nutrients: Rich in protein, fiber, vitamins, and minerals. Low in sodium and saturated fat.

Prep Time: 30 minutes

8. Vegan Chili

Ingredients:

1 can black beans, drained and rinsed

1 can kidney beans, drained and rinsed

1 can diced tomatoes

1 bell pepper, diced

1 onion, diced

2 cloves garlic, minced

1 tablespoon chili powder

1 teaspoon cumin

Salt and pepper to taste

Instructions:

Add the onion and garlic to a large pot and sauté until softened

Add bell pepper, chili powder, and cumin. Cook for 2-3 minutes.

Stir in diced tomatoes, black beans, and kidney beans.

Simmer for 20- 25 minutes, stirring occasionally.

To taste, add salt and pepper for seasoning.

Serve hot, garnished with chopped cilantro or sliced green onions if desired.

Nutrients: High in fiber, protein, vitamins, and minerals. Low in sodium and saturated fat.

Prep Time: 40 minutes

9. Vegan Buddha Bowl

Ingredients:

1 cup cooked quinoa

Assorted vegetables (roasted sweet potatoes, steamed broccoli, sliced avocado)

1/4 cup hummus

2 tablespoons tahini

Juice of 1 lemon

Salt and pepper to taste

Instructions:

Arrange cooked quinoa and assorted vegetables in a bowl.

In a small bowl, whisk together hummus, tahini, lemon juice, salt, and pepper to make the dressing.

Drizzle dressing over the Buddha bowl.

Serve immediately.

Nutrients: Balanced with protein, fiber, vitamins, and minerals. Low in sodium and saturated fat.

Prep Time: 30 minutes

10. Vegan Lentil Sloppy Joes

Ingredients:

1 cup lentils, rinsed

1 onion, diced

2 cloves garlic, minced

1 bell pepper, diced

1 can crushed tomatoes

2 tablespoons tomato paste

1 tablespoon maple syrup

1 tablespoon apple cider vinegar

1 teaspoon chili powder

Salt and pepper to taste

Whole wheat burger buns (optional)

Instructions:

Add the onion and garlic to a large pot and sauté until softened

Add bell pepper and cook for another 2-3 minutes.

Stir in lentils, crushed tomatoes, tomato paste, maple syrup, apple cider vinegar, chili powder, salt, and pepper.

Bring to a simmer and cook for 25-30 minutes, until lentils are tender.

Serve hot on whole wheat burger buns, if desired.

Nutrients: High in fiber, protein, vitamins, and minerals. Low in sodium and saturated fat.

Prep Time: 40 minutes

CHAPTER 7

Poultry, Meat and Lamb Recipes

Introduction:

The DASH (Dietary Approaches to Stop Hypertension) diet is a dietary approach aimed at lowering blood pressure and promoting heart health. Incorporating lean meats like poultry, meat, and lamb into your DASH diet can provide essential nutrients while helping you maintain a healthy blood pressure. Here are 10 delicious and healthy DASH diet recipes featuring poultry, meat, and lamb.

1. Grilled Lemon Herb Chicken:

Ingredients:

Boneless, skinless chicken breasts

Fresh lemon juice

Olive oil

Garlic cloves

Roughly chopped herbs (parsley, thyme, rosemary, etc.)

Salt and pepper to taste

Instructions:

Combine the lemon juice, olive oil, chopped herbs, minced garlic, salt, and pepper in a bowl.

For a minimum of half an hour, marinate chicken breasts in the marinade

Preheat grill to medium-high heat.

Cook the chicken for 6 to 8 minutes on each side, or until it's done

Serve hot with a side of steamed vegetables or a fresh salad.

Nutrients: High in protein, low in saturated fat.

Prep Time: 40 minutes.

2. Turkey and Quinoa Stuffed Bell Peppers:

Ingredients:

Ground turkey

Quinoa

Bell peppers

Onion

Garlic

Tomato sauce

Italian seasoning

Low-sodium chicken broth

Low-fat shredded cheese (optional)

Instructions:

Preheat oven to 375°F (190°C).

Cook quinoa according to package instructions.

In a skillet, cook ground turkey with onion and garlic until browned.

Add cooked quinoa, tomato sauce, Italian seasoning, and chicken broth to the skillet. Cook until heated through.

Remove the seeds and cut off the tops of the bell peppers.

Stuff each bell pepper with the turkey-quinoa mixture.

Stuffed peppers should be put on a baking dish, covered with foil, and baked for twenty to thirty minutes.

Optionally, sprinkle shredded cheese on top of stuffed peppers and bake uncovered for an additional 5 minutes.

Serve hot.

Nutrients: High in protein, fiber, and vitamins.

Prep Time: 45 minutes.

3. Herb-Crusted Baked Salmon:

Ingredients:

Salmon fillets

Whole wheat bread crumbs

Fresh herbs (such as dill, parsley, and chives)

Lemon zest

Olive oil

Salt and pepper to taste

Instructions:

Preheat oven to 400°F (200°C).

In a food processor, pulse bread crumbs, herbs, lemon zest, olive oil, salt, and pepper until combined.

Arrange the salmon fillets on a parchment paper-lined baking pan

Press the herb mixture onto the top of each salmon fillet.

Bake in the preheated oven for 12-15 minutes or until salmon is cooked through.

Serve hot with a side of roasted vegetables or brown rice.

Nutrients: Rich in omega-3 fatty acids, protein, and antioxidants.

Prep Time: 20 minutes.

4. Mediterranean Lamb Skewers:

Ingredients:

Lamb cubes

Cherry tomatoes

Red onion

Bell peppers

Olive oil

Lemon juice

Garlic

Oregano

Salt and pepper to taste

Instructions:

Combine the olive oil, lemon juice, oregano, minced garlic, salt, and pepper in a bowl

Thread lamb cubes onto skewers alternating with cherry tomatoes, onion slices, and bell peppers.

Brush skewers with the olive oil mixture.

Preheat grill to medium-high heat.

Grill skewers for 10-12 minutes, turning occasionally, until lamb is cooked to desired doneness.

Serve hot with a side of Greek salad and whole wheat pita bread.

Nutrients: High in protein, vitamins, and minerals.

Prep Time: 30 minutes.

5. Lean Beef Stir-Fry:

Ingredients:

Lean beef strips

Vegetable mixtures (including broccoli, snap peas, and bell peppers)

Low-sodium soy sauce

Garlic

Ginger

Olive oil

Brown rice (optional)

Instructions:

Heat the olive oil in a wok or big skillet over medium-high heat

Add minced garlic and ginger, stir-fry for 30 seconds.

Add beef strips and cook until browned.

Add mixed vegetables and stir-fry until tender-crisp.

Pour in low-sodium soy sauce and cook for an additional 2-3 minutes.

Serve hot over brown rice if desired.

Nutrients: High in protein, fiber, and antioxidants.

Prep Time: 25 minutes.

6. Chicken and Vegetable Skewers with Yogurt Sauce:

Ingredients:

Chicken breast, cut into chunks

Cherry tomatoes

Zucchini, sliced

Red onion, cut into chunks

Olive oil

Lemon juice

Garlic powder

Paprika

Salt and pepper to taste

Greek yogurt

Cucumber, diced

Fresh dill, chopped

Lemon zest

Instructions:

Olive oil, lemon juice, paprika, garlic powder, salt, and pepper should all be combined in a bowl.

Toss chicken chunks, cherry tomatoes, zucchini, and red onion in the mixture.

Thread marinated chicken and vegetables onto skewers.

Preheat grill to medium-high heat. Grill skewers for 10-12 minutes, turning occasionally, until chicken is cooked through and vegetables are tender.

In a small bowl, mix Greek yogurt, diced cucumber, fresh dill, lemon zest, salt, and pepper to make the yogurt sauce.

Serve grilled chicken and vegetable skewers with yogurt sauce on the side.

Nutrients: High in protein, vitamins, and probiotics.

Prep Time: 30 minutes.

7. Turkey Meatball Lettuce Wraps:

Ingredients:

Ground turkey

Onion, finely chopped

Garlic, minced

Egg

Whole wheat breadcrumbs

Italian seasoning

Salt and pepper to taste

Lettuce leaves

Tomato, diced

Avocado, sliced

Fresh cilantro, chopped

Instructions:

Preheat oven to 375°F (190°C).

In a bowl, mix ground turkey, chopped onion, minced garlic, egg, breadcrumbs, Italian seasoning, salt, and pepper until well combined.

Shape the mixture into meatballs and place them on a baking sheet lined with parchment paper.

Meatballs should be baked for 20 to 25 minutes, or until well done, in a preheated oven

Arrange lettuce leaves on a plate. Place turkey meatballs on top of the lettuce leaves.

Garnish with diced tomato, sliced avocado, and chopped cilantro.

Serve immediately.

Nutrients: High in protein, fiber, and healthy fats.

Prep Time: 35 minutes.

8. Grilled Lemon Herb Lamb Chops:

Ingredients:

Lamb chops

Fresh lemon juice

Olive oil

Garlic cloves, minced

Fresh rosemary, chopped

Fresh thyme leaves

Salt and pepper to taste

Instructions:

Lemon juice, olive oil, minced garlic, chopped thyme, chopped rosemary, and salt and pepper should all be combined in a bowl

Marinate lamb chops in the mixture for at least 1 hour.

Preheat grill to medium-high heat.

Grill lamb chops for 3-4 minutes per side for medium-rare, or adjust cooking time according to desired doneness.

Serve hot with a side of roasted vegetables or quinoa.

Nutrients: High in protein, iron, and vitamins.

Prep Time: 1 hour 10 minutes (including marination time).

9. Balsamic Glazed Chicken Breasts:

Ingredients:

Chicken breasts

Balsamic vinegar

Honey

Garlic, minced

Dijon mustard

Olive oil

Salt and pepper to taste

Instructions:

In a small saucepan, combine balsamic vinegar, honey, minced garlic, Dijon mustard, olive oil, salt, and pepper.

Bring the mixture to a simmer over medium heat and cook until slightly thickened, stirring occasionally.

Preheat grill to medium-high heat.

After adding salt and pepper to the chicken breasts, grill them for 6 to 8 minutes on each side, or until they are cooked through

Brush the grilled chicken breasts with the balsamic glaze and serve hot.

Nutrients: High in protein, antioxidants, and flavor.

Prep Time: 25 minutes.

10. Beef and Vegetable Kebabs with Chimichurri Sauce:

Ingredients:

Beef sirloin, cut into cubes

Bell peppers, cut into chunks

Red onion, cut into chunks

Olive oil

Garlic, minced

Red wine vinegar

Fresh parsley, chopped

Fresh cilantro, chopped

Red pepper flakes

Salt and pepper to taste

Instructions:

In a bowl, mix olive oil, minced garlic, red wine vinegar, chopped parsley, chopped cilantro, red pepper flakes, salt, and pepper to make the chimichurri sauce.

Thread beef cubes, bell peppers, and red onion onto skewers.

Preheat grill to medium-high heat. Grill kebabs for 8-10 minutes, turning occasionally, until beef is cooked to desired doneness and vegetables are tender.

Serve hot with chimichurri sauce drizzled over the top.

Nutrients: High in protein, vitamins, and antioxidants.

Prep Time: 35 minutes.

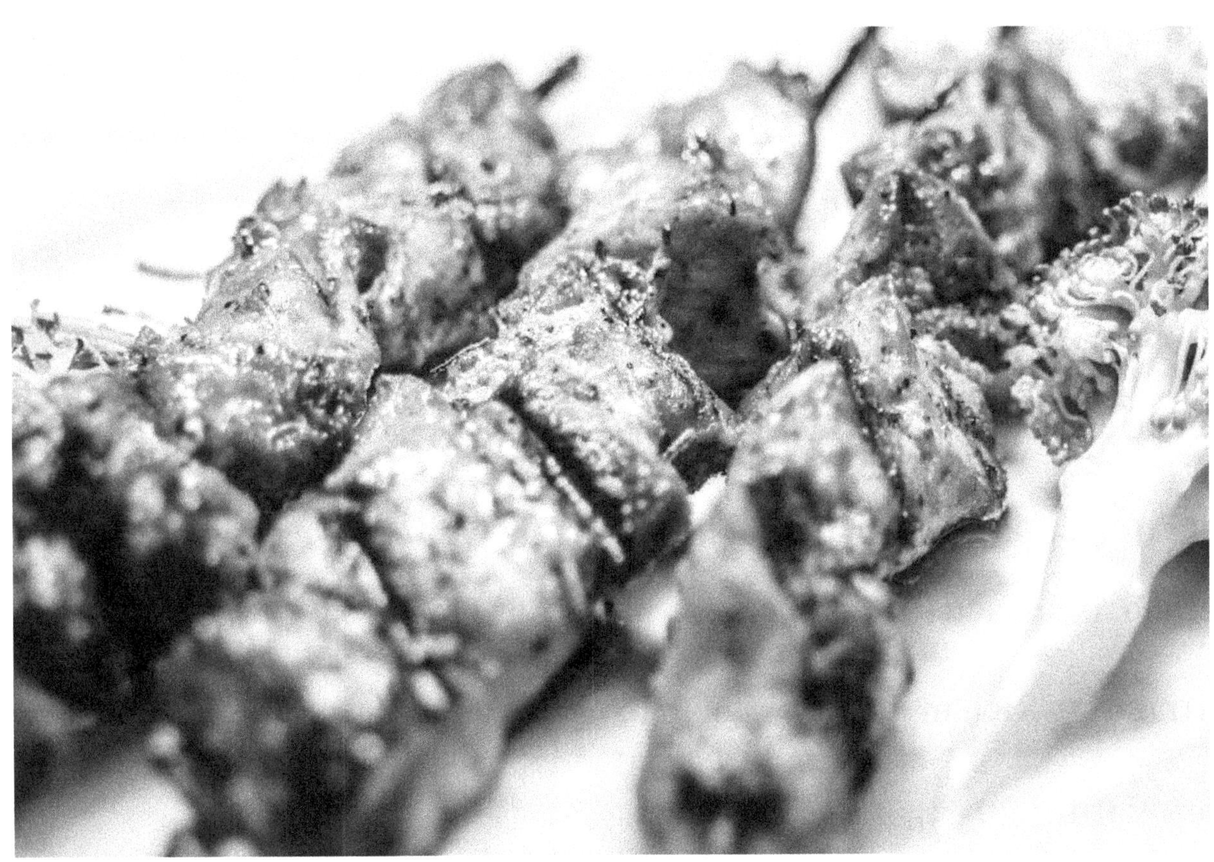

CHAPTER 8

Sauce, Stew and Soup Recipes

Introduction to DASH Diet:

The DASH (Dietary Approaches to Stop Hypertension) diet is designed to lower blood pressure and promote heart health by emphasizing fruits, vegetables, whole grains, lean proteins, and low-fat dairy while minimizing sodium, saturated fats, and processed foods.

Here are 10 healthy DASH diet sauce, stew, and soup recipes to support lower blood pressure and overall heart health:

Mediterranean Tomato Sauce:

Ingredients: Tomatoes, garlic, olive oil, onions, basil, oregano, salt, pepper.

Instructions: Sauté onions and garlic in olive oil. Stir in the diced tomatoes, oregano, basil, and salt and pepper. Simmer until thickened.

Nutrients: Rich in lycopene, vitamin C, and antioxidants.

Prep Time: 20 minutes.

Quinoa Vegetable Stew:

Ingredients: Quinoa, carrots, celery, onions, bell peppers, vegetable broth, tomatoes, spinach.

Instructions: Sauté onions, carrots, celery, and bell peppers. Add quinoa, tomatoes, vegetable broth, and simmer until quinoa is cooked. Stir in spinach.

Nutrients: High in fiber, vitamins, and minerals.

Prep Time: 30 minutes.

Lentil Soup:

Ingredients: Lentils, carrots, celery, onions, garlic, vegetable broth, cumin, paprika.

Instructions: Sauté onions, garlic, carrots, and celery. Add lentils, vegetable broth, cumin, paprika, and simmer until lentils are tender.

Nutrients: High in fiber, protein, and iron.

Prep Time: 40 minutes.

Roasted Red Pepper Sauce:

Ingredients: Red bell peppers, garlic, olive oil, basil, salt, pepper.

Instructions: Roast peppers until charred. Peel off skin and blend with garlic, olive oil, basil, salt, and pepper until smooth.

Nutrients: Rich in vitamin C, antioxidants, and healthy fats.

Prep Time: 25 minutes.

Minestrone Soup:

Ingredients: Cannellini beans, tomatoes, carrots, celery, onions, zucchini, spinach, vegetable broth, whole wheat pasta.

Instructions: Sauté onions, carrots, celery, and zucchini. Add tomatoes, vegetable broth, beans, and pasta. Simmer until pasta is cooked. Stir in spinach.

Nutrients: Packed with fiber, protein, and vitamins.

Prep Time: 45 minutes.

Tahini Lemon Sauce:

Ingredients: Tahini, lemon juice, garlic, water, salt.

Instructions: Whisk tahini, lemon juice, garlic, water, and salt until smooth.

Nutrients: Good source of healthy fats, vitamin C, and minerals.

Prep Time: 10 minutes.

Vegetable Barley Stew:

Ingredients: Barley, carrots, potatoes, onions, garlic, vegetable broth, thyme, bay leaves.

Instructions: Sauté onions, garlic, carrots, and potatoes. Add barley, vegetable broth, thyme, bay leaves, and simmer until barley is tender.

Nutrients: High in fiber, vitamins, and minerals.

Prep Time: 50 minutes.

Ginger Carrot Soup:

Ingredients: Carrots, ginger, onions, garlic, vegetable broth, coconut milk, turmeric.

Instructions: Sauté onions, garlic, and ginger. Add carrots, vegetable broth, turmeric, and simmer until carrots are soft. Blend with coconut milk until smooth.

Nutrients: Rich in beta-carotene, antioxidants, and anti-inflammatory properties.

Prep Time: 35 minutes.

Cilantro Lime Dressing:

Ingredients: Cilantro, lime juice, garlic, olive oil, honey, salt.

Instructions: Blend cilantro, lime juice, garlic, olive oil, honey, and salt until well combined.

Nutrients: Packed with vitamin C, antioxidants, and healthy fats.

Prep Time: 15 minutes.

Black Bean Soup:

Ingredients: Black beans, onions, garlic, bell peppers, tomatoes, cumin, chili powder, vegetable broth.

Instructions: Sauté onions, garlic, and bell peppers. Add black beans, tomatoes, vegetable broth, cumin, chili powder, and simmer until flavors meld.

Nutrients: High in fiber, protein, and antioxidants.

Prep Time: 40 minutes.

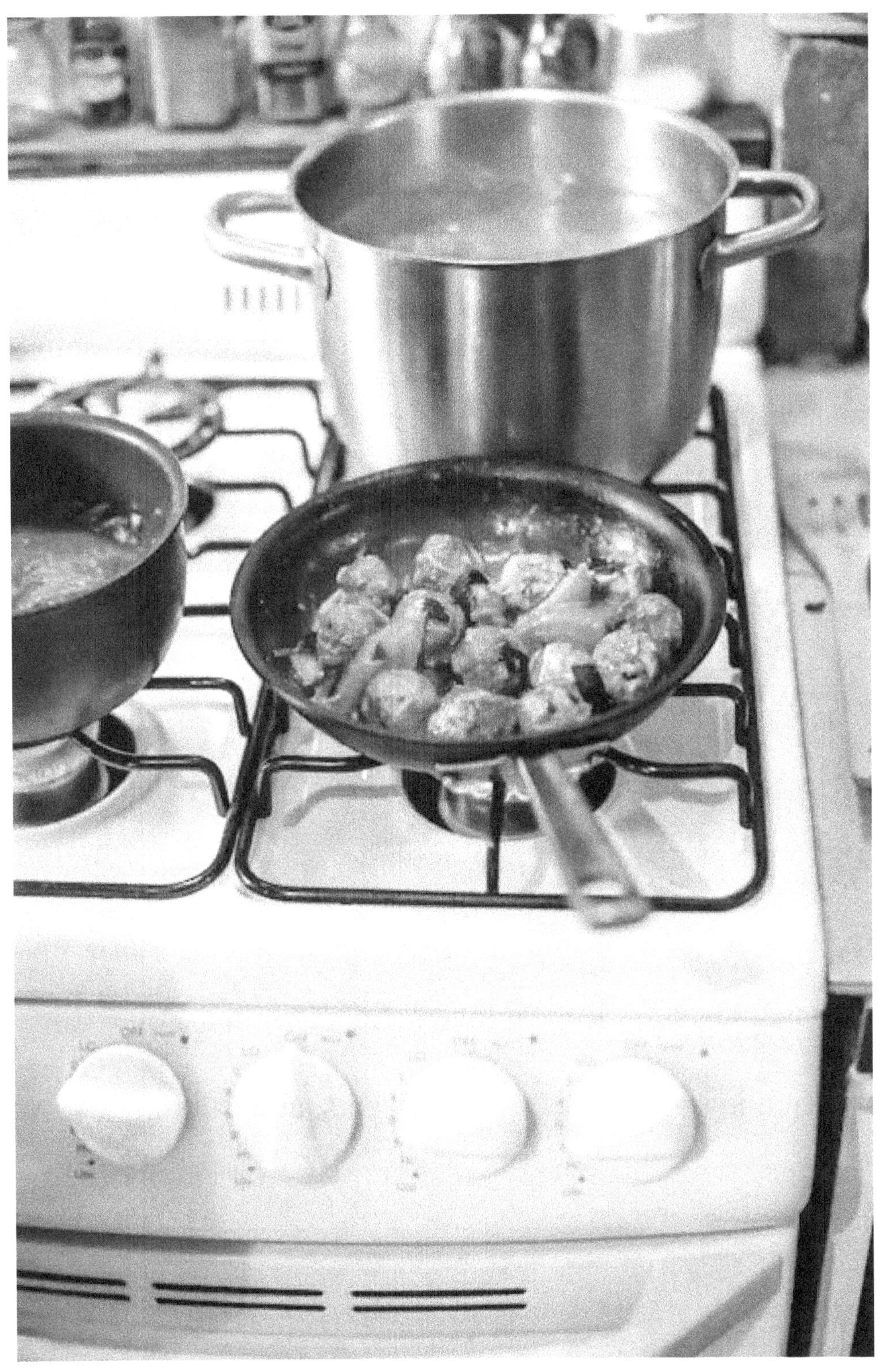

CHAPTER 9

Desserts, Snacks and Smoothies Recipes

Introduction:

Maintaining a healthy heart and managing blood pressure is essential for overall well-being. The DASH (Dietary Approaches to Stop Hypertension) diet emphasizes consuming fruits, vegetables, lean proteins, and whole grains while limiting saturated fats, sweets, and sodium. Here are 10 delicious dessert, snack, and smoothie recipes aligned with the DASH diet to support heart health.

1. Berry Yogurt Parfait

Ingredients: Greek yogurt, mixed berries (strawberries, blueberries, raspberries), honey or maple syrup, granola.

Instructions: Layer Greek yogurt, berries, and granola in a glass. Drizzle with honey or maple syrup. Repeat layers. Serve chilled.

Nutrients: Rich in protein, fiber, antioxidants, and calcium.

Prep Time: 5 minutes.

2. Avocado Chocolate Mousse

Ingredients: Ripe avocado, cocoa powder, honey or agave syrup, vanilla extract.

Instructions: Blend avocado, cocoa powder, honey or agave syrup, and vanilla extract until smooth. Chill before serving.

Nutrients: High in healthy fats, fiber, and antioxidants.

Prep Time: 10 minutes.

3. Cucumber and Hummus Snack

Ingredients: Cucumber slices, hummus.

Instructions: Spread hummus on cucumber slices. Serve as a refreshing snack.

Nutrients: Rich in fiber, vitamins, and minerals, and low in calories.

Prep Time: 5 minutes.

4. Apple Nachos

Ingredients: Apple slices, almond butter, dark chocolate chips, chopped nuts, shredded coconut.

Instructions: Arrange apple slices on a plate. Drizzle with almond butter and sprinkle with chocolate chips, nuts, and coconut.

Nutrients: Provides fiber, healthy fats, and antioxidants.

Prep Time: 10 minutes.

5. Banana-Oat Energy Bites

Ingredients: Mashed ripe bananas, rolled oats, almond butter, honey, cinnamon.

Instructions: Mix all ingredients in a bowl. Roll into small balls. Refrigerate until firm.

Nutrients: High in fiber, potassium, and protein.

Prep Time: 15 minutes.

6. Spinach and Berry Smoothie

Ingredients: Spinach, mixed berries, banana, Greek yogurt, almond milk.

Instructions: Blend all ingredients until smooth. If necessary, thin the consistency with almond milk.

Nutrients: Packed with antioxidants, vitamins, and calcium.

Prep Time: 5 minutes.

7. Frozen Yogurt Bark

Ingredients: Greek yogurt, honey, granola, sliced almonds, dried fruit.

Instructions: Mix yogurt and honey. Spread onto a baking sheet. Sprinkle with granola, almonds, and dried fruit. Once frozen firm, break into pieces.

Nutrients: High in protein, calcium, and fiber.

Prep Time: 10 minutes + freezing time.

8. Peach and Cottage Cheese Bowl

Ingredients: Sliced peaches, cottage cheese, honey, cinnamon.

Instructions: Arrange peach slices and cottage cheese in a bowl. Sprinkle with cinnamon and drizzle with honey.

Nutrients: Provides protein, calcium, and vitamins.

Prep Time: 5 minutes.

9. Carrot Cake Oatmeal Cookies

Ingredients: Rolled oats, grated carrots, raisins, cinnamon, nutmeg, honey.

Instructions: Mix all ingredients in a bowl. Form into cookies and bake until golden brown.

Nutrients: Rich in fiber, beta-carotene, and antioxidants.

Prep Time: 20 minutes.

10. Green Tea Smoothie

Ingredients: Green tea, spinach, pineapple chunks, banana, honey.

Instructions: Brew green tea and let it cool. Blend with spinach, pineapple, banana, and honey until smooth.

Nutrients: Loaded with antioxidants, vitamins, and minerals.

Prep Time: 10 minutes.

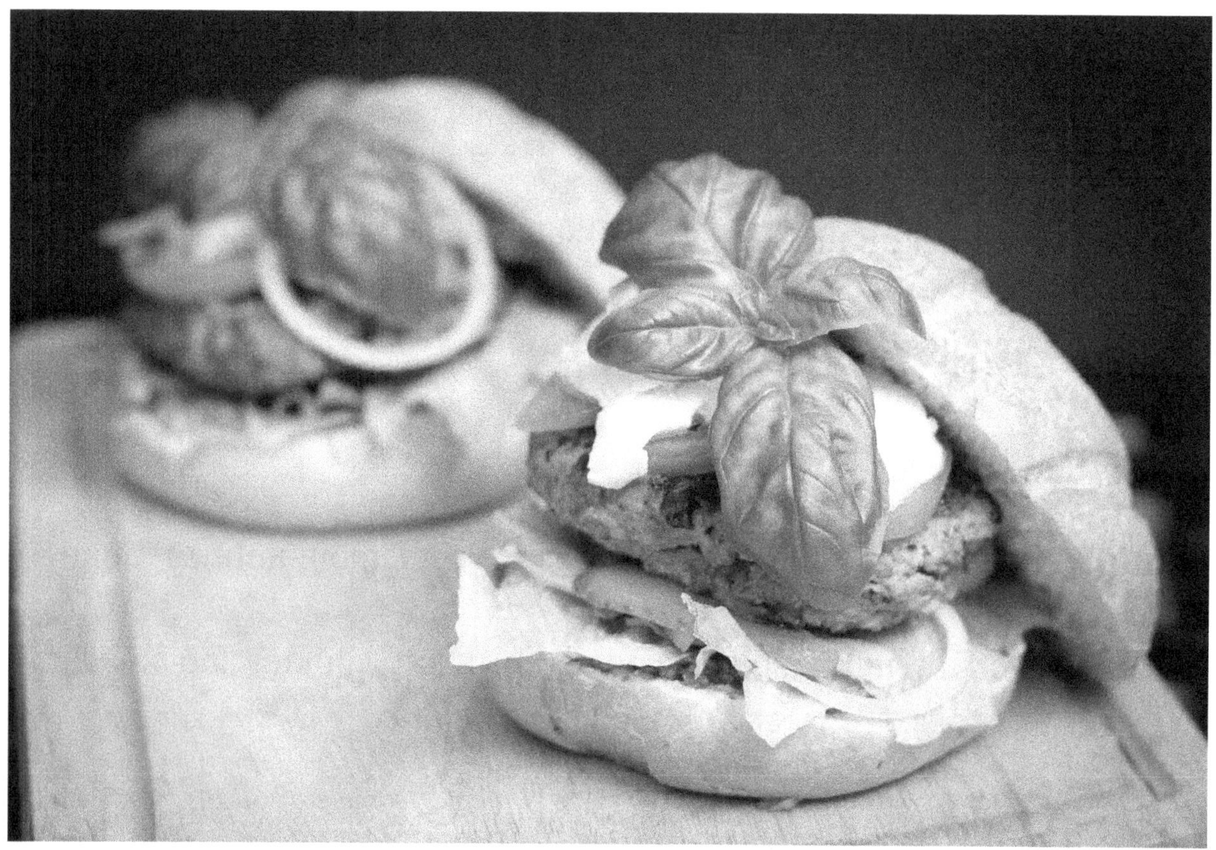

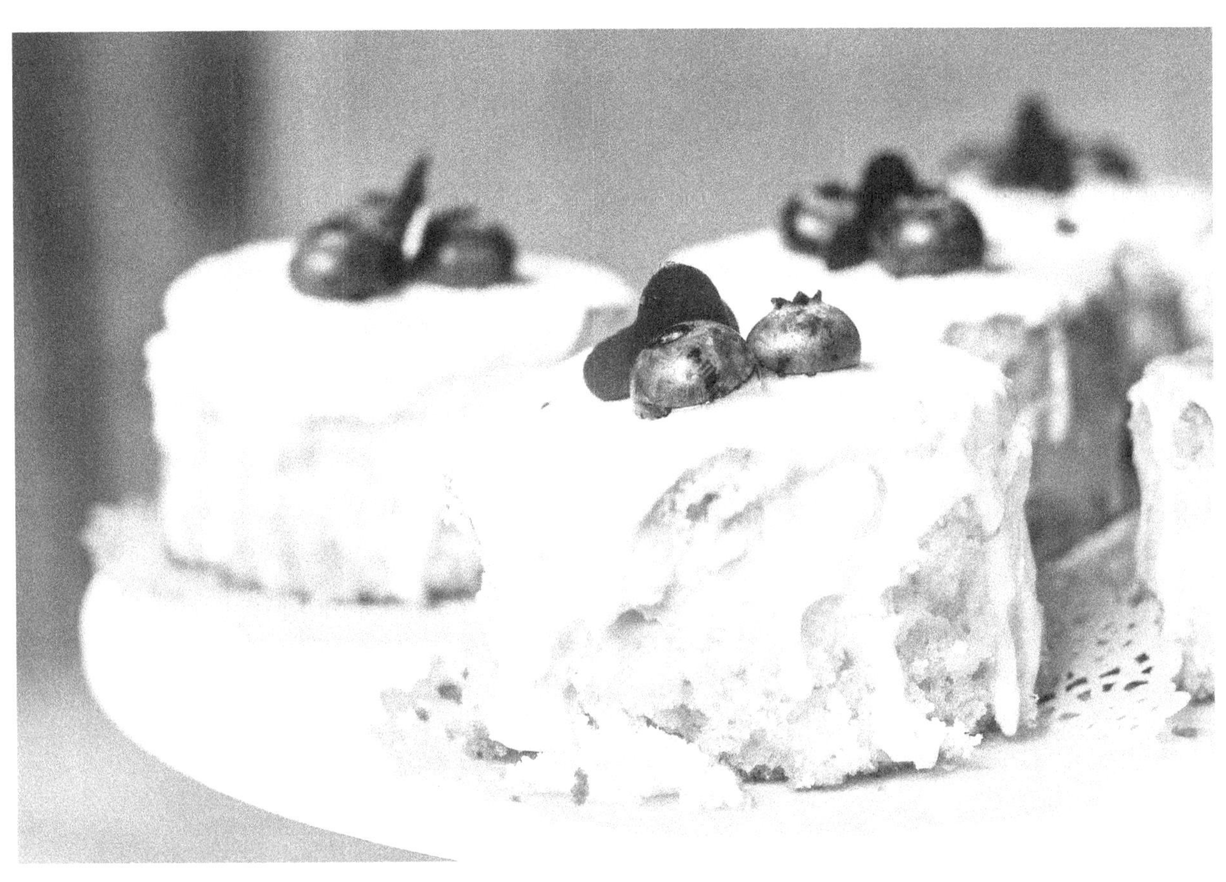

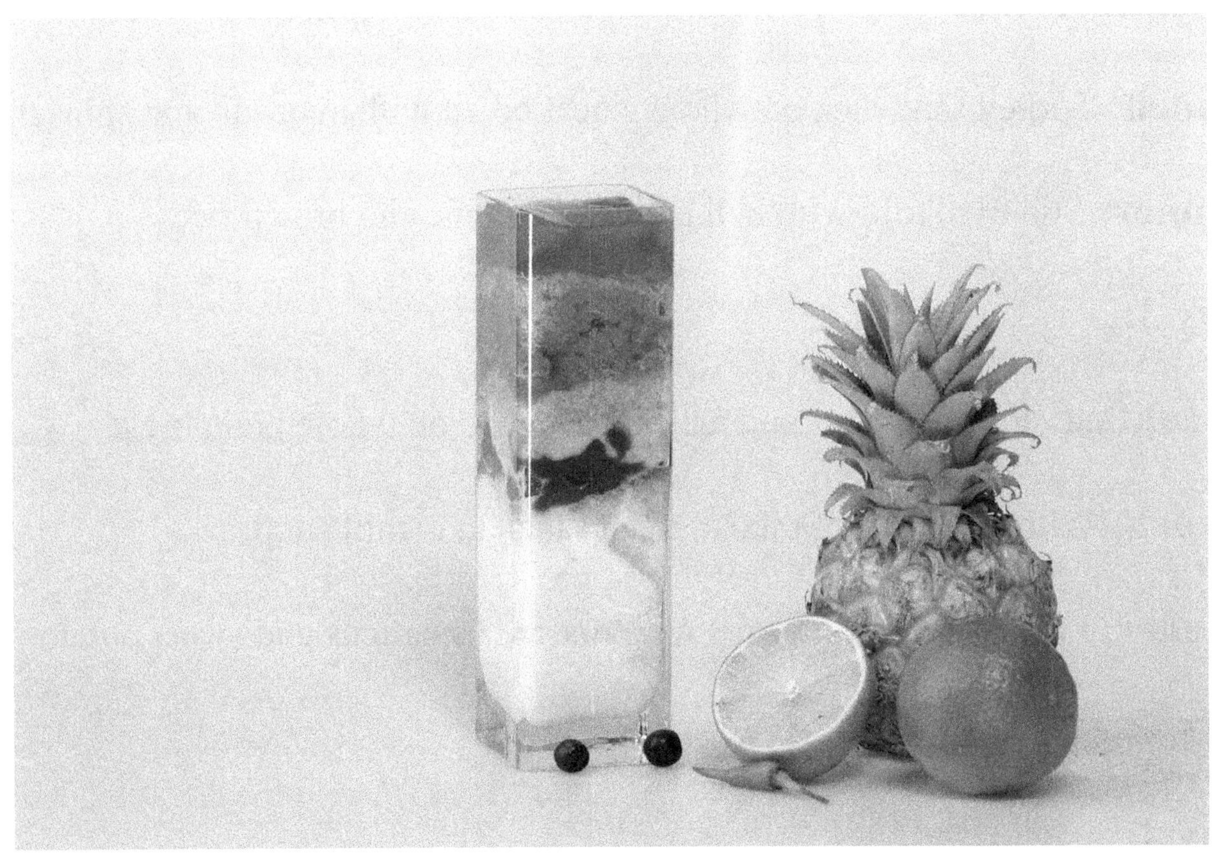

CHAPTER 10

30 Days Dash Diet Meal Plan

Day 1:

Breakfast: Oatmeal with berries and almonds

Lunch: Grilled chicken salad with mixed greens, tomatoes, cucumbers, and olive oil vinaigrette

Dinner: Quinoa and steamed broccoli with baked salmon

Day 2:

Breakfast: Greek yogurt with sliced bananas and a sprinkle of walnuts

Lunch: Turkey sandwich on whole wheat bread with avocado and spinach

Dinner: Stir-fried tofu with bell peppers, onions, and brown rice

Day 3:

Breakfast: Poached eggs and mashed avocado on whole grain bread

Lunch: With a serving of mixed green salad and lentil soup

Dinner: Grilled shrimp skewers with roasted asparagus and sweet potato

Day 4:

Breakfast: Smoothie made with spinach, pineapple, banana, and almond milk

Lunch: Quinoa salad dressed with lime vinaigrette, black beans, corn, and cherry tomatoes

Dinner: Grilled chicken breast with sautéed spinach and whole wheat pasta

Day 5:

Breakfast: Slicked strawberries and whole grain cereal with skim milk

Lunch: Veggie wrap with hummus, shredded carrots, cucumbers, and lettuce

Dinner: Roasted Brussels sprouts, wild rice, and baked fish

Day 6:

Breakfast: Cottage cheese topped with sliced peaches and a drizzle of honey

Lunch: Chickpea salad with diced bell peppers, cucumbers, tomatoes, and feta cheese

Dinner: Turkey meatballs with marinara sauce over whole wheat spaghetti

Day 7:

Breakfast: Whole wheat English muffin with scrambled eggs and spinach

Lunch: Quinoa-stuffed bell peppers with a side of mixed greens

Dinner: Grilled steak with roasted cauliflower and mashed sweet potatoes

Day 8:

Breakfast: Whole grain pancakes topped with fresh berries and a drizzle of honey

Lunch: Spinach and feta omelet served with a side of whole grain toast

Dinner: Baked chicken breast with roasted vegetables (such as carrots, zucchini, and bell peppers) and quinoa

Day 9:

Breakfast: Smoothie bowl made with mixed berries, spinach, Greek yogurt, and a sprinkle of granola

Lunch: Tuna salad made with canned tuna, mixed greens, cherry tomatoes, olives, and a light vinaigrette

Dinner: Grilled shrimp and vegetable kebabs served with brown rice

Day 10:

Breakfast: Avocado toast on whole grain bread topped with cherry tomatoes and a poached egg

Lunch: Mediterranean salad with chickpeas, cucumbers, red onion, feta cheese, and a lemon-herb vinaigrette

Dinner: Baked salmon with steamed green beans and quinoa pilaf

Day 11:

Breakfast: Greek yogurt parfait with layers of yogurt, sliced bananas, and granola

Lunch: A side of healthy grain bread is given with the lentil and vegetable soup.

Dinner: Turkey chili topped with chopped green onions and a side of steamed broccoli

Day 12:

Breakfast: Whole grain waffles topped with sliced strawberries and a dollop of Greek yogurt

Lunch: Hummus and veggie wrap with shredded carrots, bell peppers, cucumbers, and lettuce

Dinner: Grilled chicken Caesar salad with homemade dressing and whole grain croutons

Day 13:

Breakfast: Veggie scramble made with eggs, spinach, bell peppers, and onions served with whole grain toast

Lunch: Quinoa salad with black beans, corn, cherry tomatoes, avocado, and lime vinaigrette

Dinner: Roasted Brussels sprouts, wild rice, and baked fish

Day 14:

Breakfast: Overnight oats made with rolled oats, almond milk, chia seeds, and topped with sliced bananas and almonds

Lunch: Caprese salad with fresh mozzarella, tomatoes, basil, and a drizzle of balsamic glaze

Dinner: Brown rice with mixed vegetables with stir-fried tofu

Day 15:

Breakfast: Whole grain toast topped with mashed avocado, sliced tomatoes, and a sprinkle of feta cheese

Lunch: Salad of quinoa and grilled veggies with a lemon-tahini sauce

Dinner: Grilled lemon-herb chicken breast with roasted cauliflower and brown rice

Day 16:

Breakfast: Smoothie made with spinach, pineapple, Greek yogurt, and a spoonful of almond butter

Lunch: With lettuce, tomato, and a whole grain tortilla, a turkey and avocado wrap

Dinner: Baked halibut with roasted asparagus and quinoa

Day 17:

Breakfast: Greek yogurt with honey, sliced almonds, and fresh berries

Lunch: Lentil and kale salad with roasted sweet potatoes, goat cheese, and a balsamic vinaigrette

Dinner: Stir-fried shrimp with mixed vegetables served over whole wheat noodles

Day 18:

Breakfast: Slicing bananas with whole grain cereal with skim milk

Lunch: Chickpea and vegetable stir-fry with a side of brown rice

Dinner: Grilled sirloin steak with sautéed mushrooms and a baked sweet potato

Day 19:

Breakfast: Whole wheat English muffin with scrambled eggs, spinach, and feta cheese

Lunch: Quinoa tabbouleh salad with cucumber, cherry tomatoes, parsley, and lemon dressing

Dinner: Baked chicken thighs with roasted Brussels sprouts and quinoa pilaf

Day 20:

Breakfast: Cottage cheese topped with sliced peaches and a sprinkle of cinnamon

Lunch: Veggie burger on a whole grain bun with lettuce, tomato, and avocado

Dinner: Baked salmon with steamed green beans and wild rice

Day 21:

Breakfast: Pancakes made with whole grains, mixed berries, and maple syrup drizzled over them

Lunch: Greek salad with mixed greens, olives, tomatoes, cucumbers, feta cheese, and a light vinaigrette

Dinner: Turkey meatballs in marinara sauce served over whole wheat spaghetti

Day 22:

Breakfast: Whole grain toast topped with scrambled eggs, sautéed spinach, and cherry tomatoes

Lunch: Quinoa and black bean salad with diced bell peppers, corn, avocado, and lime-cilantro dressing

Dinner: Grilled tofu with stir-fried broccoli, bell peppers, and brown rice

Day 23:

Breakfast: Smoothie bowl made with mixed berries, spinach, Greek yogurt, and a sprinkle of granola

Lunch: Mediterranean wrap with grilled chicken, hummus, cucumber, tomato, and lettuce in a whole wheat tortilla

Dinner: Baked cod with roasted Brussels sprouts and quinoa pilaf

Day 24:

Breakfast: Greek yogurt parfait with layers of yogurt, sliced bananas, and granola

Lunch: Lentil soup with a side of mixed green salad topped with cherry tomatoes, cucumbers, and a light vinaigrette

Dinner: Turkey chili served with a side of steamed broccoli

Day 25:

Breakfast: Whole grain waffles topped with sliced strawberries and a dollop of Greek yogurt

Lunch: Hummus and veggie sandwich on whole grain bread with shredded carrots, bell peppers, cucumber, and spinach

Dinner: Grilled shrimp skewers with roasted asparagus and quinoa

Day 26:

Breakfast: Veggie scramble made with eggs, bell peppers, onions, and spinach served with whole grain toast

Lunch: Quinoa salad with chickpeas, diced tomatoes, cucumbers, feta cheese, and a lemon-herb vinaigrette

Dinner: Baked chicken breast with sautéed kale and wild rice

Day 27:

Breakfast: Overnight oats made with rolled oats, almond milk, chia seeds, and topped with sliced peaches and almonds

Lunch: Caprese salad with fresh mozzarella, tomatoes, basil, and a drizzle of balsamic glaze

Dinner: Brown rice with mixed vegetables with stir-fried tofu

Day 28:

Breakfast: Whole grain toast topped with mashed avocado, sliced tomatoes, and a poached egg

Lunch: Spinach and feta omelet served with a side of whole grain toast

Dinner: Grilled lemon-herb chicken breast with roasted cauliflower and quinoa

Day 29:

Breakfast: Whole grain pancakes topped with fresh berries and a drizzle of honey

Lunch: With lettuce, tomato, and a whole grain tortilla, a turkey and avocado wrap

Dinner: Baked halibut with roasted asparagus and quinoa

Day 30:

Breakfast: Smoothie made with spinach, pineapple, Greek yogurt, and a spoonful of almond butter

Lunch: Lentil and kale salad with roasted sweet potatoes, goat cheese, and a balsamic vinaigrette

Dinner: Grilled sirloin steak with sautéed mushrooms and a baked sweet potato

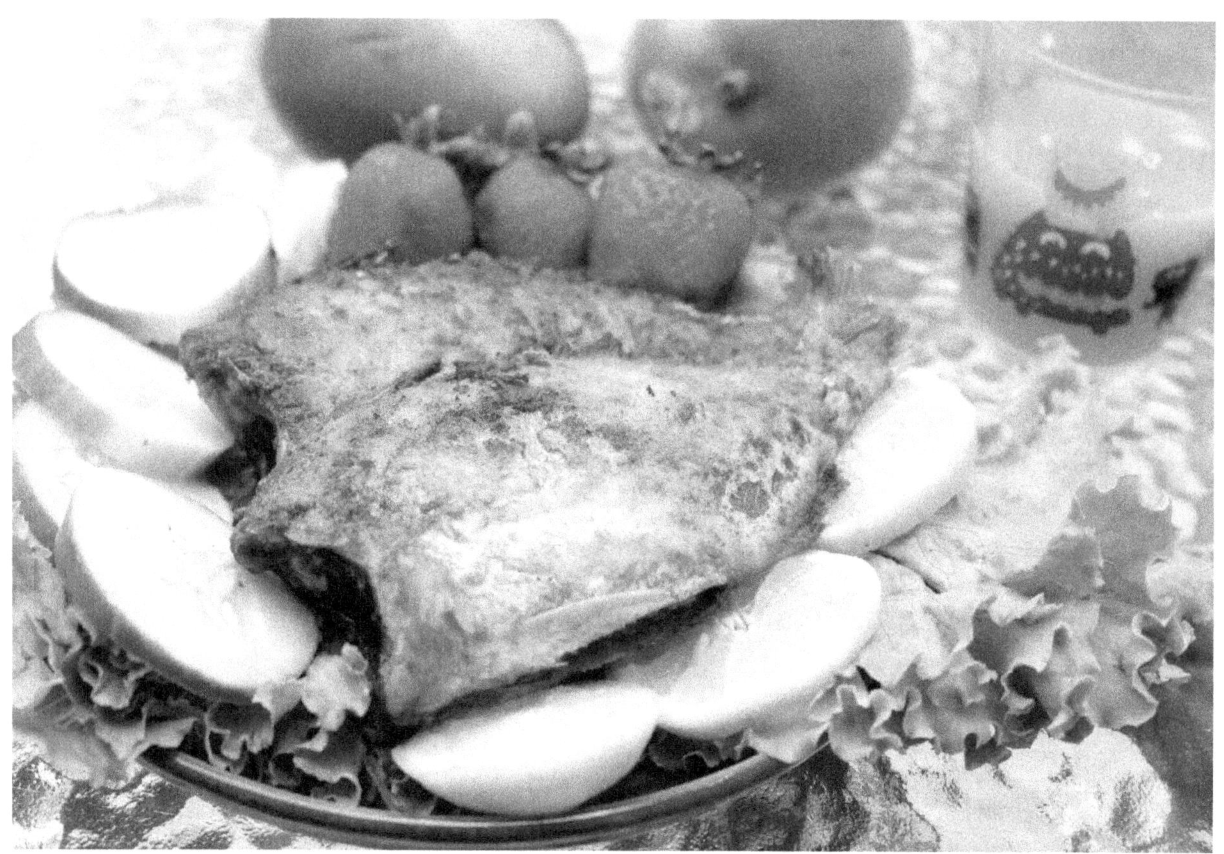

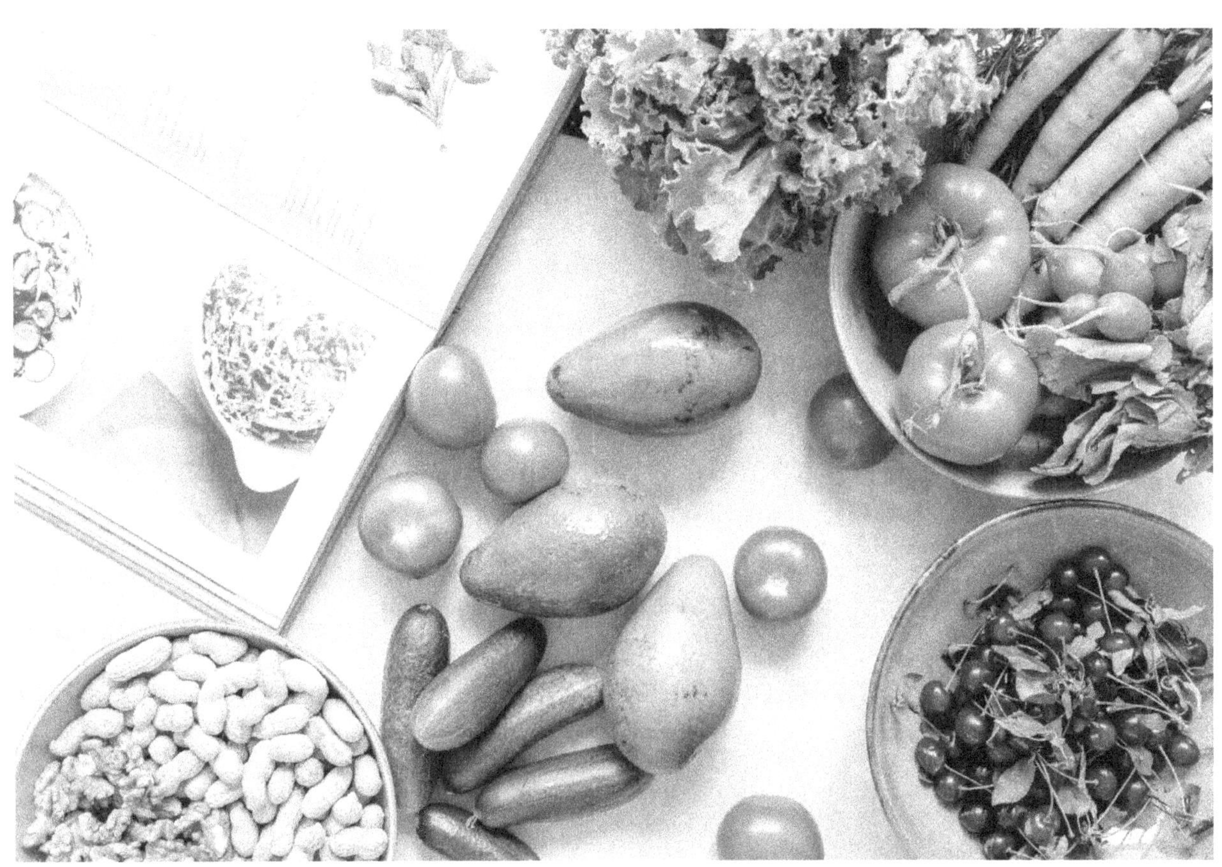

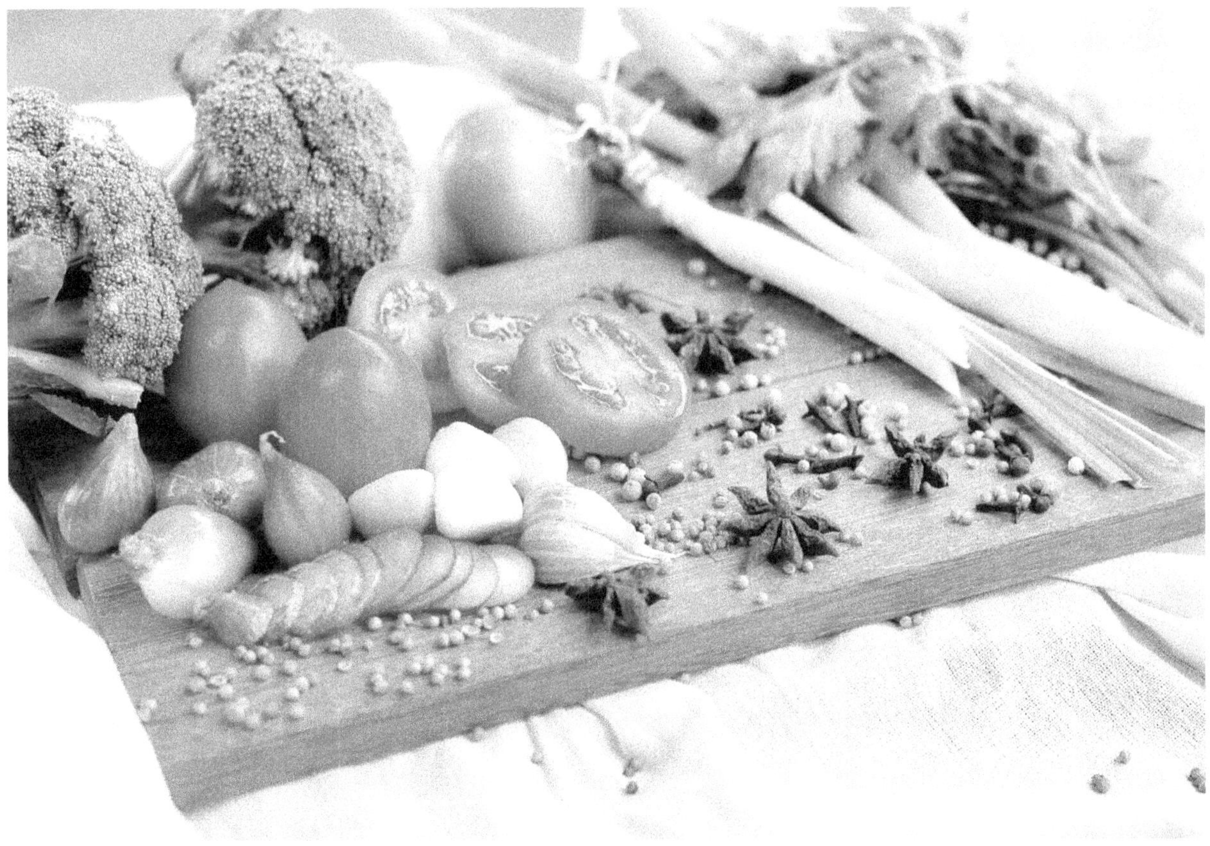

CHAPTER 11

Healthy Fruits

Introduction:

Maintaining a healthy blood pressure and promoting heart health are essential for overall well-being. Incorporating nutrient-rich fruits into your diet can be a delicious and effective way to achieve these goals. Here are ten fruits known for their ability to lower blood pressure and support heart health, along with instructions on how to incorporate them into your diet, their key nutrients, and preparation times.

Bananas

Instructions: Enjoy bananas sliced on top of oatmeal or yogurt, blended into smoothies, or eaten as a convenient on-the-go snack.

Nutrients: Rich in potassium, which helps regulate blood pressure, and fiber, which supports heart health.

Prep Time: Instant (peeling required)

Oranges

Instructions: Eat oranges as a refreshing snack, juice them for a hydrating beverage, or incorporate them into salads for a burst of citrus flavor.

Nutrients: High in vitamin C, antioxidants, and fiber, which can help lower blood pressure and reduce the risk of heart disease.

Prep Time: Instant (peeling required)

Apples

Instructions: Slice apples and pair them with nut butter for a satisfying snack, bake them into desserts, or add them to salads for a crunchy texture.

Nutrients: Packed with fiber, antioxidants, and flavonoids, which promote heart health and lower blood pressure.

Prep Time: Instant (washing and slicing required)

Berries (Blueberries, Strawberries, Raspberries)

Instructions: Enjoy berries fresh as a snack, add them to yogurt or cereal, blend them into smoothies, or use them as toppings for pancakes or waffles.

Nutrients: Rich in antioxidants, vitamins, and fiber, which help reduce inflammation, lower blood pressure, and improve heart health.

Prep Time: Instant (washing required)

Avocados

Instructions: Mash avocados onto toast, add them to salads or sandwiches, blend them into smoothies, or use them as a creamy base for dips and sauces.

Nutrients: High in monounsaturated fats, potassium, and fiber, which support healthy cholesterol levels and lower blood pressure.

Prep Time: Instant (peeling and slicing required)

Kiwi

Instructions: Peel and slice kiwi for a refreshing snack, add it to fruit salads or yogurt, blend it into smoothies, or use it as a colorful garnish for desserts.

Nutrients: Loaded with vitamin C, potassium, and fiber, which contribute to heart health and blood pressure regulation.

Prep Time: Instant (peeling and slicing required)

Pomegranate

Instructions: Enjoy pomegranate seeds as a tangy snack, sprinkle them on salads or oatmeal, blend them into juices or smoothies, or use them as a garnish for savory dishes.

Nutrients: Rich in antioxidants, vitamins, and potassium, which help lower blood pressure and improve heart health.

Prep Time: Moderate (extracting seeds can take a few minutes)

Watermelon

Instructions: Slice watermelon into wedges for a hydrating snack, blend it into refreshing juices or smoothies, or add it to fruit salads for a burst of sweetness.

Nutrients: High in water content, vitamins, and antioxidants, which contribute to hydration, lower blood pressure, and overall heart health.

Prep Time: Instant (slicing required)

Grapes

Instructions: Enjoy grapes as a convenient snack, freeze them for a refreshing treat, add them to salads or cheese plates, or blend them into juices or smoothies.

Nutrients: Packed with antioxidants, vitamins, and resveratrol, which support heart health and may help lower blood pressure.

Prep Time: Instant (washing required)

Pears

Instructions: Slice pears and enjoy them on their own or paired with cheese, add them to salads or oatmeal, bake them into desserts, or blend them into smoothies.

Nutrients: High in fiber, vitamins, and antioxidants, which promote heart health and may help regulate blood pressure.

Prep Time: Instant (washing and slicing required)

CONCLUSION

Embarking on a journey towards a healthier lifestyle often begins with dietary choices, and the DASH (Dietary Approaches to Stop Hypertension) diet stands as a beacon of evidence-based guidance for those seeking to improve their cardiovascular health and overall well-being.

As we've explored throughout this cookbook tailored for beginners, the principles of the DASH diet emphasize the consumption of nutrient-rich foods, particularly fruits, vegetables, lean proteins, whole grains, and dairy products with reduced fat content, while reducing consumption of sodium, saturated fats, and added sugars.

The DASH diet not only offers a practical approach to reducing high blood pressure but also serves as a comprehensive framework for promoting heart health and preventing chronic diseases such as cardiovascular disease and diabetes.

By focusing on whole foods that are naturally rich in vitamins, minerals, antioxidants, and fiber, individuals can enjoy a varied and flavorful diet that supports optimal health from within.

Through the recipes and guidelines provided in this cookbook, beginners can discover the versatility and deliciousness of DASH-friendly meals, whether they're whipping up a vibrant salad bursting with colorful fruits and vegetables, savoring a hearty bowl of whole grain pasta with lean protein and marinara sauce, or indulging in a refreshing fruit smoothie as a satisfying snack.

Furthermore, the DASH diet emphasizes not just what to eat but also how to eat, encouraging mindful eating practices such as paying attention to hunger and fullness cues, savoring each bite, and enjoying meals in a relaxed environment.

By fostering a positive relationship with food and prioritizing nourishment over restriction, individuals can cultivate sustainable dietary habits that support long-term health and well-being.

As beginners embark on their DASH diet journey, it's important to remember that progress is achieved through consistency, patience, and a willingness to explore new flavors and ingredients.

By gradually incorporating DASH-approved recipes into their meal rotation, individuals can gradually transition to a healthier eating pattern without feeling overwhelmed or deprived.

In essence, this cookbook serves as a valuable resource and companion for those embarking on their DASH diet journey, providing practical tips, flavorful recipes, and evidence-based guidance to support their pursuit of better health.

Whether you're seeking to lower your blood pressure, improve your heart health, or simply adopt a more balanced approach to eating, the DASH diet offers a roadmap towards a healthier, happier life. So, let's embrace the power of wholesome ingredients, nourishing meals, and mindful eating as we journey towards optimal health and vitality together.

MEAL PLANNER

Weekly Meal Planner

	BREAKFAST	LUNCH	DINNER	SNACKS
MON				
TUE				
WED				
THU				
FRI				
SAT				
SUN				

Note :

Shopping list

Weekly Meal Planner

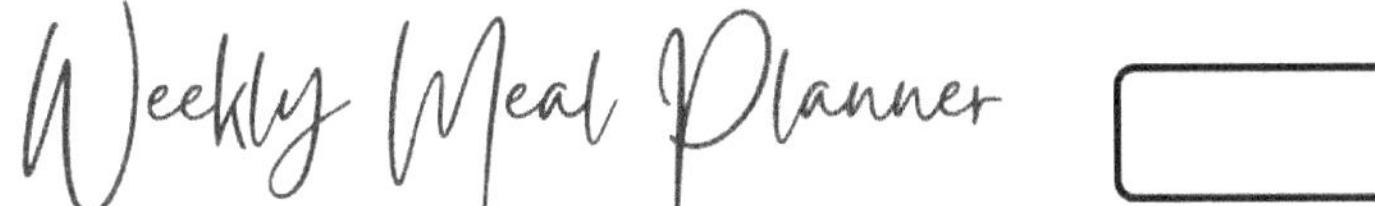

	BREAKFAST	LUNCH	DINNER	SNACKS
MON				
TUE				
WED				
THU				
FRI				
SAT				
SUN				

Note :

Shopping list

Weekly Meal Planner

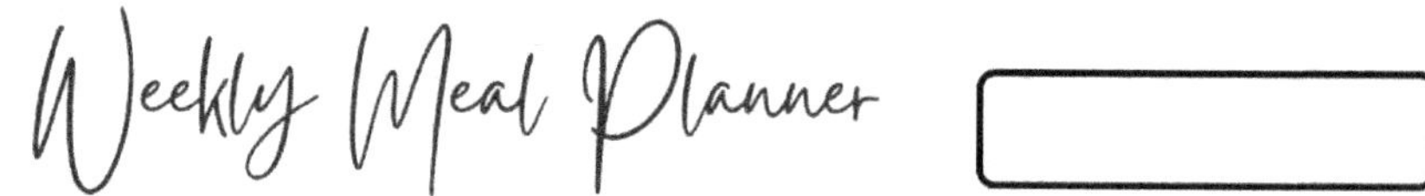

	BREAKFAST	LUNCH	DINNER	SNACKS
MON				
TUE				
WED				
THU				
FRI				
SAT				
SUN				

Note :

Shopping list

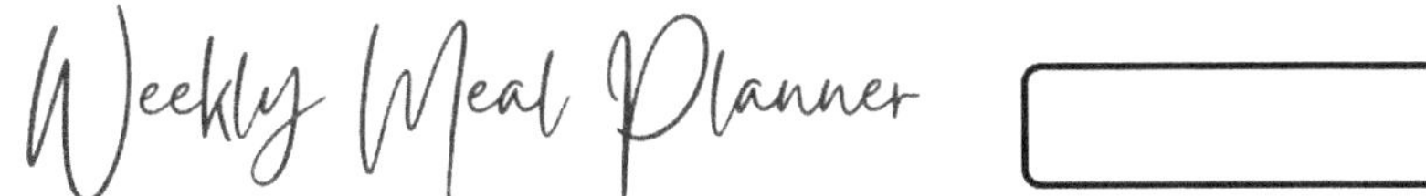

	BREAKFAST	LUNCH	DINNER	SNACKS
MON				
TUE				
WED				
THU				
FRI				
SAT				
SUN				

Note :

Shopping list

Weekly Meal Planner

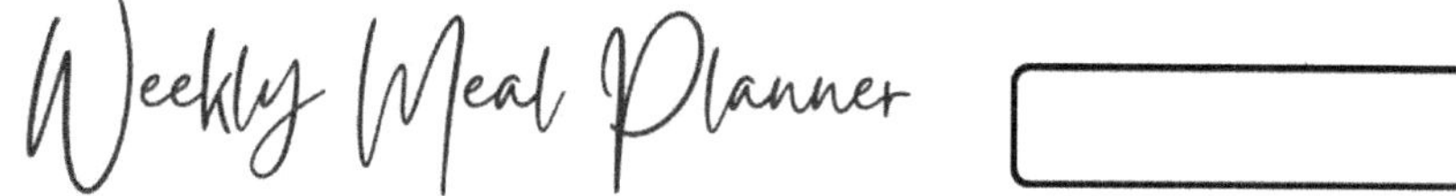

	BREAKFAST	LUNCH	DINNER	SNACKS
MON				
TUE				
WED				
THU				
FRI				
SAT				
SUN				

Note :

Shopping list

I have a request

Dear readers, I hope you enjoy this book, please try possible and gives this book feedback

If you are in need of additional information, question or enquiries about all these recipes, ask through this

Catherinedietinfo@gmail.com